Copyright © Yoga Satsanga Ashram UK 2018

Written by
Yogachariya Jnandev

Editor
Yogacharini Deepika Saini

ISBN 978-1-9995850-0-6

First Published June 2018

Designed, Printed & Published by Design Marque

Printed in Great Britain by www.designmarque.co.uk

Material within this book, including text and images, is protected by copyright. It may not be copied, reproduced, republished, downloaded, posted, broadcast or transmitted in any way except for your own personal, non-commercial use. Prior written consent of the copyright holder must be obtained for any other use of material. Copyright in all materials and/or works comprising or contained within this book remains with Author and other copyright owner(s) as specified. No part of this book may be distributed or copied for any commercial purpose.

YOGA
Questions & Answers

by
Yogachariya Jnandev Giri

About Yogachariya Jnandev Giri
(Surender Kumar Saini)

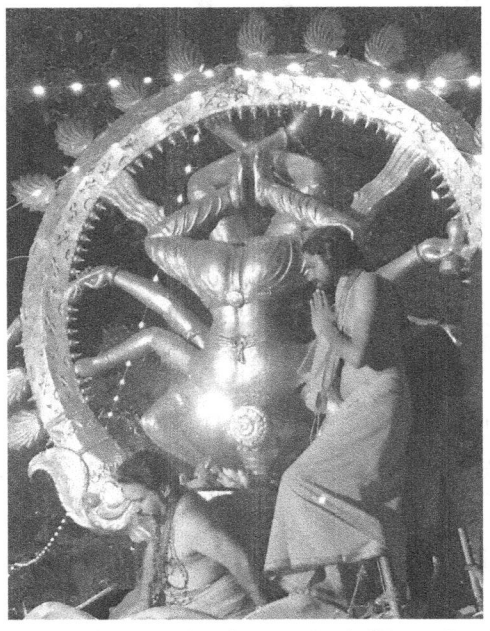

Yogachariya Jnandev with Dr Ananda Balayogi at Kambali Swami Temple, Puducherry

Yogachariya Jnandev Giri was born in a traditional Hindu family in Khetri, Rajasthan, India. Yoga, Hinduism and Spiritualism was part of his life practically since birth.

Jnandev met with many great Yogis, Sadhus and Monks from various traditions or lineages. Even though he first started Hatha Yoga when he was 17-18 years old, but he studied the main scriptures Mahabharta, Ramayana, Yoga Sutras and others under his Grandfathers guidance as he was a Bhajan writer, singer and Satsang leader in the local community travelling around that part of Rajasthan.

Jnandevs academic background began training as a pharmacist, which he practiced for a short period quickly realising it was not his destiny, he then graduated in maths, physics and chemistry as he always had a strong interest in science. During this time his interest in yoga meditation and samadhi grew deeper which lead him to seek out a Msc in Yoga and meditation.

Jnandev enrolled in the Msc in yoga and Preksha meditation in 2000-2002 at Jain Vishwa Bharti Ladnun University, Rajisthan. Here he spent most of his time with the Jain monks along with his academic studies. This University has one of the most well-re sourced libraries in India, with many original manuscripts where Jnandev was able to study very old scripts in Sanskrit. Due to his unusual focus on learning he was allowed special access to all the sections of the library thanks to blessings of one of his many Gurus Samami Sthita Prajna, where he spent most of his free time. Jnandev completed this course as the top-students/gold medallist awarded in the presence of President of India, Abdul Kalam Azad at that time.

After his M.Sc. he began working as a Yoga Teacher at Maheshwari Girls Public School (MGPS), Vidyadhar Nagar, Jaipur. Here he taught Yoga classes and moral science to 2,600 girls every week. During this time, he based himself in Yoga Satsanga Ashram, Jaipur under guidance of Swami Mahaveer Nath and took diksha later on to become a Saddhu. He was given the name Swami Ananta Nath. During these years he visited many ashrams and travelled around Northen India and learnt Yoga and Adhyatm (spiritualism).

After working in the school for 3 years he left to find silence and live in solitude to grow further in his yoga sadhana for some time, living in some forest parts of N. India before eventually making his way to the Tamil Nadu region South of India.

In 2006 Jnandev found Ananda Ashram, International Centre for Yoga Education and Research (ICYER) Pondicherry and he met with Ammaji Meenakshi Devi Bhavanani September 2006 and he still feels a lot of gratitude for giving him her time to meet and accept him onto the 6-month intensive International Yoga Teacher Training course. Jnandev found the course to be life transforming and the most comprehensive, scientifically balanced and authentic type of trainings that can be found in India today. This course follows the ancient teachings of classical yoga which has today been disseminated into many yoga paths or styles. In traditional ashrams the Guru-chela system is really the only way to learn holistic and authentic Yoga though initiation into a Paramparai, although this is highly challenging for Ahamkaras and Asmita (negative ego and i-ness).

Then in 2007 a friendship developed between Jnandev and Deepika who was also on the same course at ICYER. In January 2008 with the blessings of Jnandevs family they got married in Jaipur. Consequently, Jnandev had to leave the Ashram system and follow the householder life, which he is very grateful for a very different opportunity to learn grow and practice. In December of 2008 they had their first son Siddha and now have two more Mahadev and Krishna.

In 2008 Jnandev came to live in the UK with Deepika and together they founded Yoga Satsanga Ashram, Wales UK. In 2010 they began teacher training courses after being approached by some local students. Since then the Ashram and the courses have expanded.

Presently Jnandev leads Yoga Teacher training courses 200 hours, 300 hours, 500 hours, children's yoga teacher training and aids Deepika in Pregnancy Yoga Teacher Training. Work on a 1000 hours advanced training and yoga Therapy courses are in progress. In addition to this Jnandev teaches weekly classes and has run several workshops for those with mental or physical disabilities under Arts Care Wales. Jnandev also runs community classes for Pembrokshire County council to help get Yoga out as much as possible to the people who need it most.

Jnandev has also written 5 other books, produced a DVD and a CD to help the yoga practitioner or teacher.

Dedication and Thanks

I dedicate this work to all our sincere yoga students, Yoga family and my wife Yogacharini Deepika Saini for their true desire to learn through some true enquiries, which motivated me to put these questions and answers together the best I can. I would like to offer my deep love and gratitude to all the masters of yoga who have shown me light on the path. I am truly grateful for all the love, guidance and support I have received from Ammaji Meenakshi Devi Bhavanani and Dr Ananda Balayogi Bhavanani, at ICYER.

This book is for all those yoga seekers, Sadhakas and Sadhakis, Yoga Instructors and Yoga Teachers who would desire to know about some of the common terms used in Yoga. Please remember this is just to put seeds in our mind and heart, to know and understand these concepts we need in-depth study and sadhana on each of these subjects.

Yogachariya Jnandev Giri
Founder and Director, Yoga Satsanga Ashram, Wales, UK

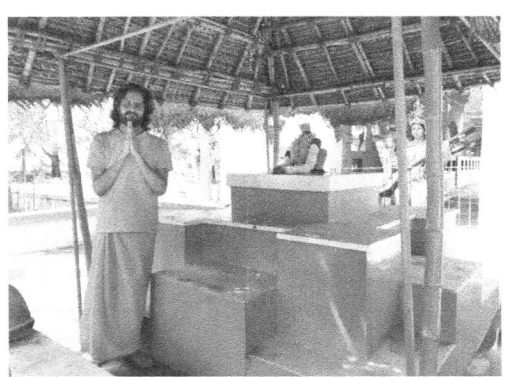

Yogachariya Jnandev at Swami Dr Gitananda Giriji Samadhi, Kambali Swami Temple, Puducherry

CONTENTS

Blessings 16
Yogacharya Dr. Ananda Balayogi Bhavanani 17
Yoga: The Ideal Way Of Life 19
Claiming One's Birthright Through Yoga 32
What is the traditional meaning of Yoga? 42
Why should one Practice Yoga? 42
Is yoga goal or a path? 43
Where is the Origin of Yoga? 43
What is Hinduism? 43
What are Chatur Dharmas or Ashrams? 43
What are Chatura Yugas? 44
What are Vedas? 44
What are four Vedas? 45
Is Yoga part of Hinduism? 45
Do I Have to be a Hindu to Practice Yoga? 46
How does yoga evolve through various ages from Satayuga to Kaliyuga? .. 46
What is Raja Yoga? 47
What is Bahiranga and Antaranga Yoga? 48
What are Eight Limbs of Raja Yoga? 48
What is Hatha Yoga? 48
What is Karma Yoga? 49
What is Mantra Yoga? 49
What is Tantra Yoga? 50
What is Jnana Yoga? 50
What is Dhyana Yoga? 51
What is Kriya Yoga? 52
What is Pranayama Yoga? 52
What is Kundalini Yoga? 52
What are the Seven Chakras? 53
Do the Chakras exist in Physical Body? 54
What are the Pancha-Koshas? 55
What is Pranayama Kosha? 55
What are the Naris? 55
How are the Chakras associated with Nadis? 56
Is there a connection between Chakras and Nerve Plexus? 57
How would we associate Chakras with Endocrine System? 58
What is Parampara or Lineage? 59
What is Bhakti Yoga? 60
What is Swara Yoga? 61
What are Key Yoga Scriptures? 61

- Yoga Sutras ... 62
- Who was Patanjali? ... 63
- Bhagavata Gita ... 64
- Yoga Vashistha ... 65
- Shiva Samhita ... 66
- Yoga Chudamani ... 67
- Vijnana Bhairava Tantra ... 68
- Shiva Swarodaya ... 69
- Hatha Yoga Pradipika ... 69
- Gheranda Samhita ... 71
- Yajnavalkya Samhita ... 72
- What are the original dates of Yoga Scriptures? ... 73
- What is the Four Yugas?. ... 73
- Indian Mythological History and Scriptures ... 74
- Did only men practice yoga as we hear from many modern yoga teachers? 75
- Did ascetics or spiritual seekers only practice yoga? ... 76
- What is an Ashram? ... 76
- Is it true that first Hatha Yoga was taught in 1918 in India? ... 76
- What are Eight Limbs of Yoga in Summary? ... 77
- Yama ... 77
- Niyama ... 77
- Asana ... 77
- Pranayama ... 77
- Pratyahara ... 78
- Dharna ... 78
- Dhyana ... 78
- Samadhi ... 78
- What is Yama? ... 78
- What are Pancha Yamas? ... 79
- Ahimsa ... 79
- Satya ... 79
- Asteya ... 79
- Brahmachariya ... 80
- Aparigraha ... 80
- What are the Panch Niyamas? ... 80
- Shaucha ... 80
- Samtosha ... 81
- Tapah ... 81
- Swadhyaya ... 81
- Isvara Pranidhana ... 82
- Do I need to practice Yamas and Niyamas Universally? ... 82
- What are Shata Karmas? ... 82
- What is Asana? ... 83

Why do we Practice Asana?	83
How does Asana helps dealing with stress?	83
What is Vinyasa or Kriya in Hatha Yoga?	84
What does Suriya Namaskar mean?	84
How many Classical Asanas are there?	84
Yoga in Modern Age	85
What is Pranayama?	85
What is Prana?	85
What are the Pancha Vayus?	86
What are the associations of Pancha Vayus with Chakras?	87
Is Pranayama Breathing exercise?	87
Why do we practice Pranayama?	87
Pranayama according to Ammaji Meenakshi Devi Bhavanani	88
What are four aspects of Pranayama?	88
What is classical Pranayamas according to Hatha Yoga Pradipika?	89
Shitakari Pranayama	89
Shitali Pranayama	89
Bhramari Pranayama	89
Bhastrika Pranayama	90
Murcha Pranayama	90
Suriya Bhedana	91
Ujjayi Pranayama	91
Plavini Pranayama	92
Dr Swami Gitananda Giri Ji on Pranayama	92
How in depth is Hatha Yoga Science in Gitananda Tradition according to Ammaji Meenakshi Devi?	92
Is there the connection between mind and prana?	93
What is the success in Pranayama?	93
What is Pratyahara?	94
Is Pratyahara Bahiranga or Antaranga Yoga?	94
What are senses?	94
What are five Jnanendriyas?	95
What are five Karmendriyas?	95
What are other three subtle sense organs?	95
How to practice Pratyahara?	96
What is Dharna?	96
How can breath be used a Dharna?	97
What is Samayama Yoga?	97
What is Dhyana?	97
How important is Meditation to attain Samadhi?	98
Can I Practice Dhyana?	98
What are three essential principals behind meditation?	98

- What is Samadhi? 99
- What are kinds or types of Samadhi? 99
- Is Yoga mystic or esoteric? 100
- Is Yoga Scientific then? 100
- What is Karma? 101
- What are types of Karma? 101
- What are the types of Karma in reference to time and fruits? 102
- Can I be free of doing Karma? 102
- How can I be free from fruits of Karma? 102
- How to know what is right and wrong in Karma? 103
- What are five fundamental Truths or reality? 103
- What are the Obstacles or Antarayas on Path of Yoga? 103
- What are Nine Obstacles? 104
- What are the four tools to remove obstacles? 104
- What are five states of mind? 105
- What are Five modifications of Mind or Pancha Vrittis? 105
- What are Pancha Kleshas or cause of suffering? 106
- What are the subtle four remedies? 106
- What is Abhyasa? 106
- What is Vairagya? 107
- What are three Gunas? 107
- What is Pancha Mahabhutas? 107
- What is Pranava? 108
- How do I chant a Mantra? 108
- What are Guru and Sadguru? 108
- How important is it to use Sanskrita in Yoga? 109
- How do I attain success in Yoga? 109
- Which are Three Bandhas? 109
- What is a mudra? 109
- Do I need to live extreme ascetic life to be successful in Yoga? 110
- Is Yoga Kriya or Akriya? 110
- Do I need to follow a particular path or lineage of Yoga? 110
- What are Avidya and Vidya? 110
- What is Satsanga? 111
- What is Kirtan? 111
- What is Bhajan? 112
- What are Puja and Aarti? 112
- What is Namaskar or Namaste? 112
- Why do we have to touch feet of a Guru or Master in Yoga? 113
- Is there a Scientific explanation of touching feet? 113
- What is Mauna? 113
- What is Vrata? 114
- What is Yoga Therapy? 114

What is Adhi-Vyadhi? ... 115
What is Moksha?. ... 116
What is a Siddhi? ... 116
What is a Yogi? ... 116
What is a Sadhu? ... 116
What is a Siddha? ... 117
Als Yoga to Control our Mind? ... 117
What is Ananda, Parmananda, and Satchidananda? ... 117
Who is Adhikari In Yoga? ... 117
What is Guru Dakshina? ... 118
What is Diksha? ... 118
What is Dvaita? ... 118
What is Advaita? ... 118
What are the few of many Classical Meanings of Yoga? ... 119
What is Naam Daan in Yoga? ... 119
What is Dharma? ... 120
How can I attain success in yoga or any other goals in life? ... 120
What is Mitahara? ... 120
Do I need to follow yoga practices extreme intensively to be successful? 120
What is Shavasana? ... 121
What is Yoga Nidra? ... 121
What are key four Asanas? ... 122
What is Ahara Vihara? ... 122
How Ahara Vihara is important for health and well-being? ... 122
What is Aura? ... 123
What is Atman -Parmatman? ... 123
What is Jiva? ... 123
What is Prakriti? ... 124
What are six key Indian Philosophies? ... 124
What is Samkhya Darshana? ... 124
What is Yoga Darshana? ... 125
What is Nyaya Darshana? ... 125
What is Vaisheshika Darshana? ... 125
What is Purva Mimamsa Darshana? ... 125
What is Vedanta Darshana? ... 126
What are six sub-schools or branches of Vedanta? ... 126
What is Isvara or Divine in Yoga? ... 126
What is Yajna or Yagya? ... 128
Why are English Sanskrita words spell differently in different texts? ... 128
What is Ahamkar? ... 128
Do I have to kill my Ego? ... 129
What is the role of Ego in our Yogic evolution? ... 129

Blessings

I am very pleased to see this new book on "Yoga: questions and answers" authored by my dear Yogachariya Jnandev (Surender Saini) and edited by my dear Yogacharini Deepika (Sally Saini). Both of them are an integral part of my Gitananda Yoga family worldwide and each time I vist them I can sense the growth happening both within as well as externally in their lives. Yoga Satsanga Ashram in Carmartenshire, Wales feels very much like a home to me and I have fond memories of my visits there as it is a joy to teach in such a Yogic atmosphere.

This book gives the sincere and dedicated seeker of Yoga a great amount of information. It contains brief answers to so many questions that often come up in the mind, but don't come out of the mouth. Often the students are shy to ask questions as they fear being rebuked, or face embarrassment and hence do not express their doubts. This book enables them to find the answers in an easy to read manner thus helping them grow better and in a more harmonious manner in their Yoga Sadhana.

It is vital that all modern seekers develop an understanding of Yoga as a conscious and evolutionary "way of life" as this is most often lost in the modern showbiz of "asana-like posture circuses" that abound. Unless one understands the transformative principles of Yoga, they will have merely the body but never understand and experience the spirit.

A special word of appreciation for the skilled artist who has so beautifully illustrated various concepts and added to the aesthetics of the book.

May the Guru Parampara continue to bless Yogachariya Jnandev, Yogacharini Deepika and their family as well as the Yoga family of the Ashram with success in their Yoga Sadhana.

May we all grow and glow in spirit through the life of Yoga, enabling each and every one to manifest their inherent divinity with joy, health and wellness.

Om Hari Om Tat Sat Om.

Yogacharya
Dr Ananda Balayogi Bhavanani
Chairman: ICYER at Ananda Ashram, Pondicherry
www.rishiculture.in

Yogacharya Dr. ANANDA BALAYOGI BHAVANANI
MBBS, ADY, DPC, DSM, PGDFH, PGDY, FIAY, MD (Alt.Med), C-IAYT

Yogacharya Dr. Ananda Balayogi Bhavanani is Director of the Centre for Yoga Therapy Education and Research (CYTER), and Professor of Yoga therapy at the Sri Balaji Vidyapeeth University, Pondicherry (www.sbvu.ac.in).

He is also Chairman of the International Centre for Yoga Education and Research at Ananda Ashram, Pondicherry, India (www.icyer.com) and Yoganjali Natyalayam, the premier institute of Yoga and Carnatic Music and Bharatanatyam in Pondicherry (www.rishiculture.in). He is son and successor of the internationally acclaimed Yoga team of Yogamaharishi Dr. Swami Gitananda Giri Guru Maharaj and Yogacharini Kalaimamani Ammaji, Smt Meenakshi Devi Bhavanani.

He is a Gold Medallist in Medical Studies (MBBS) with postgraduate diplomas in both Family Health (PGDFH) as well as Yoga (PGDY) and the Advanced Diploma in Yoga under his illustrious parents in 1991-93. A Fellow of the Indian Academy of Yoga, he has authored 19 DVDs and 23 books on Yoga as well as published more than two hundred papers, compilations and abstracts on Yoga and Yoga research in National and International Journals. His literary works have more than 1500 Citations, with an h-Index of 19 and an i10-Index of 33. In addition, he is a Classical Indian Vocalist, Percussionist, Music Composer and Choreographer of Indian Classical Dance.

In recent years he has travelled abroad 17 times and conducted invited talks, public events, workshops and retreats and been major presenter at Yoga conferences in the UK, USA, Italy, South Africa, Germany, Switzerland, Canada, Australia and New Zealand.

He is an Honorary International Advisor to the International Association of Yoga Therapists (www.iayt.org), the Australasian Association of Yoga Therapists (www.yogatherapy.org.au), the World Yoga Foundation (www.worldyogafoundation.in) and Gitananda Yoga Associations worldwide (www.rishiculture.in).

A recognized PhD guide for Yoga Therapy he was recognized as an IAYT Certified Yoga Therapist (C-IAYT) by the International Association of Yoga Therapists, USA in September 2016. It is notable that he is the first Indian to receive this honour.

He is currently member of numerous expert committees of the Ministry of AYUSH including its National Board for Promotion of Yoga and Naturopathy, Scientific Advisory Committee of CCRYN, Expert Committees for Celebration of International Yoga Day and the Yoga & Diabetes program. He is Consultant Resource Person for the WHO Collaborative Centre in Traditional Medicine (Yoga) at MDNIY, New Delhi. He is also EC member and Director Publications Committee of the Indian Yoga Association (www.yogaiya.in) and Board of Directors of the Council for Yoga Accreditation International (www.cyai.org).

YOGA: THE IDEAL WAY OF LIFE

Yogacharya Dr ANANDA BALAYOGI BHAVANANI
Chairman ICYER at Ananda Ashram, Pondicherry.
www.rishiculture.in

INTRODUCTION:

Yoga is gradually being welcomed into modern health care systems as an understanding of its multifarious benefits is gaining ground worldwide. In our haste to have it accepted into the mainstream medicare, we must not however forget that Yoga is first and foremost a spiritual science for the integrated, holistic development of the physical, mental and spiritual aspects of our being. Though the recent advancements in the field of research have given evidence that Yoga helps normalize human physiological and psychological functioning more importantly the practice of Yoga as a way of life is calming and provides a rare opportunity in our chaotic lives to leave the madness of the outside world behind and attain an inner peace by helping us to focus inwards. The World health organisation defines health as "The state of complete physical, mental and social wellbeing and not merely absence of disease or infirmity". The Yogic way of living is a vital tool that helps attain that 'state' of health. We must not forget that it is more important to have both a sense of "being" healthy as well as "feeling" healthy. Hence, the qualitative aspect of health, the spiritual nature of the human life is rightly considered more important in Yoga and other Indian systems of traditional medicine.

The Bhagavad Gita defines Yoga as equanimity at all levels which may also be taken as the perfect state of health where there is physical homeostasis and mental equanimity giving rise to a healthy harmony between the body and mind. The Hatha Yoga Pradipika, also states that "Yoga improves the health of all alike and wards off diseases of one who tirelessly practices Yoga whether they are young, old, decrepit, diseased or weak, provided they abide to the rules and regulations properly".

THE ORIGINAL MIND BODY MEDICINE:

Yoga is the original mind body medicine and is one of the greatest treasures of the unique Indian cultural heritage. As both an art and science it has a lot to offer humankind in terms of an understanding of both the human mind as well as all aspects of our multilayered existence. Yoga treats man as a multi layered, conscious being, possessing three bodies (sthula, sukshma and kaarana sharira) and being enveloped in a five layered (pancha kosha) of existence.

This ancient science of mind control as codified by Maharishi Patanjali more than 2500 years ago helps us to understand our mental processes as well as the cause - effect relations of a multitude of problems facing modern man. Modern man is the victim of stress and stress related disorders that threaten to disrupt his life totally. Yoga offers a way out of this 'whirlpool of stress' and is a wholistic solution to stress.

Yogic lifestyle, Yogic diet, Yogic attitudes and various Yogic practices help man to strengthen himself and develop positive health thus enabling him to withstand stress better. This Yogic "health insurance" is achieved by normalizing the perception of stress, optimizing the reaction to it and by releasing the pent up stress effectively through various Yogic practices. Yoga is a wholistic and integral science of life dealing with physical, mental, emotional and spiritual health of the individual and society.

A PERSONAL EVOLUTIONARY JOURNEY

Yoga is a continuous process. The whole problem with something being goal-oriented is that people think that the goal is something to be reached at the end of the journey, but it is the journey itself that is important. This entire yogic process is not what you learn and not what you achieve. Yoga is something that you "live" until your last breath, and even that last breath should be completed with awareness. You should go with the satisfaction of knowing that you have done your best. Yoga is a continuous process. It is a journey and the goal is the journey itself. Yoga is getting to know what your body can and cannot do. Yoga is watching the breath, slowing down the breath and discovering that you can have a wonderful control over your emotions when slowing

down the breath, because breath is the seat of our emotions. Yoga is not about the number of Yoga practices we do nor is it about how many times or how long we do them. It is all about how we live our life in tune with Dharma.

This is all about our evolutionary journey from the lower animal states of being to the highest divine states of being that has been beautifully described by the Sufi Saint Rumi hundreds of years ago. Rumi declared in ecstasy, "I died as a mineral to become a plant, I died as a plant to become an animal, I died as an animal to become a man, I died as a man to become an angel, I died as an angel to become a God. When was I ever the less by dying"?

Yoga is life and everything we do is Yoga. Yoga is in every second of life, Yoga is in every action you do and in every thought you have and in every emotion that you feel. For modern man in a modern setting, I feel more than anything else that Yoga is skill in action. Whatever you do, you should do with the attitude that it is to be done to the best of your ability and with total effort. I think that to have action that is skilful and yet not motivated by any desire is a model concept for modern man. I see Yoga, in its modern context, as skilful action without desire or concern about the fruits of our actions.

YOGA AND HEALTH :

Yoga understands health and well being as a dynamic continuum of human nature and not a mere 'state' to be attained and maintained. The lowest point on the continuum with the lowest speed of vibration is that of death whereas the highest point with the highest vibration is that of immortality. In between these two extremes lie the states of normal health and disease. For many, their state of health is defined as that 'state' in which they are able to function without hindrance whereas in reality, health is part of our evolutionary process towards Divinity. The lowest point on the dynamic health continuum with lowest speed of vibration may be equated with lowest forms of life and mineral matter while the highest point with highest speed of vibration may be equated with Divinity.

The Yogic concept of health and disease enables us to understand that the cause of physical disorder sprouts from the higher levels of the mind and beyond. Adhi – the disturbed mind is the cause and vyadhi – the disease is the effect manifested in the physical body. Maharishi Patanjali mentions "vyadhi" as a hindrance to the complete integration of the individual personality. He doesn't directly refer to the treatment of particular diseases as his approach is more holistic and expanded rather than analytical and limited. Patanjali prefers to 'integrate' rather than deal exclusively with individual symptoms of dis-integration. The diseases are merely gross symptoms that accompany disturbances of the mind called vikshepa which appear as duhkha (misery or pain), daurmanasya (dejection), angamejayatva (tremors) and svasaprasvasa, (disturbances in breathing). Through the Yoga life, one can control these disturbances before they become powerful enough to cause breakdown. The two-pronged attack advised by Patanjali is holistic: yama-niyama on the psychological side and asana-pranayama on the physical.

DEALING WITH OMNIPRESENT STRESS
Thousands of years ago, Yogeshwar Krishna in the Bhagavad Gita (often referred to as the bible of Yoga) taught us about the Yogic patho-psychology of stress and how through our attraction to the worldly sensory objects we cause our own destruction. These potent ancient teachings hold true even in today's world. In chapter Two (Samkhya Yoga), the pattern of behaviour (stress response) is given that ultimately leads to the destruction of man. In verse 62 Lord Krishna says, "Brooding on the objects of the senses, man develops attachment to them; from attachment (sanga or chanuraaga) comes desire (kama) and from unfulfilled desire, anger (krodha) sprouts forth." Verse 63 tells us, "From anger proceeds delusion (moha); from delusion, confused memory (smriti vibramah); from confused memory the ruin of reason and due to the ruin of reason (buddhi naaso) he perishes." In the very next verse (64), he also gives us a clue to equanimity of mind (samatvam) and how to become a person settled in that equanimity (stitha prajna) who is not affected by the opposites (dwandwa). He says, "but the disciplined yogi, moving amongst the sensory objects with all senses under control and

free from attraction (raaga) and aversion (dwesha), gains in tranquillity." According to Maharishi Patanjali, most of our problems stem from the five psycho-physiological afflictions (pancha klesha) that are inborn in each and every human being. These pancha klesha are ignorance (avidya), egoism (asmita) and our sense of needing to survive at any cost (abinivesha) as well as the attraction (raaga) to external objects and the repulsion (dwesha) to them. Ignorance (avidya) is usually the start of most problems along with the ego (asmita). Our sense of needing to survive at any cost (abinivesha) compounds it further. Both attraction (raaga) to external objects and the repulsion (dwesha) to them need to be destroyed in order to attain tranquillity as well as equanimity of emotions and the mind. Maharishi Patanjali further states that the practice of Kriya Yoga (Yoga of mental purification) consisting of tapa (disciplined effort), svadhyaya (self analysis) and ishwara pranidhana (surrender to the Divine will) is the means to destroy these five mental afflictions and attain to the state of samadhi or oneness with the supreme self or the Divine.

The regular practice of yogasana, kriya, mudra, bandha and pranayama helps to recondition the physical (annamaya kosha) and energy (pranamaya kosha) bodies. The practice of pratyahara, dharana and dhyana techniques helps to recondition the mind body (manomaya kosha) apparatus. All of these Yogic practices help to foster a greater mind-emotions-body understanding and bring about the union and harmony of body, emotions and mind. This righteous (right-use-ness) union is Yoga in its truest sense.

Yoga helps us to take the right attitude towards our problems and thus tackle them in an effective manner. "To have the will (iccha shakti) to change (kriya shakti) that which can be changed, the strength to accept that which can not he changed, and the wisdom (jnana shakti) to know the difference" is the attitude that needs to the cultivated. An attitude of letting go of the worries, the problems and a greater understanding of our mental process helps to create a harmony in our body, and mind whose disharmony is the main cause of 'aadi – vyadhi' or psychosomatic disorders.

PRODUCING POSITIVE HEALTH AND WELL BEING

According to Swami Kuvalayananda, founder of Kaivalyadhama positive health does not mean mere freedom from disease but is a jubilant and energetic way of living and feeling that is the peak state of well being at all levels – physical, mental, emotional, social and spiritual. He says that one of the aims of Yoga is to encourage positive hygiene and health through development of inner natural powers of body and mind. In doing so, Yoga gives special attention to various eliminative processes and reconditions inherent powers of adaptation and adjustment of body and mind. Thus, the development of positive powers of adaptation and adjustment, inherent to the internal environment of man, helps him enjoy positive health and not just mere freedom from disease. He emphasizes that Yoga produces nadi shuddhi (purification of all channels of communication) and mala shuddhi (eradication of factors that disturb balanced working of body and mind).

According to Swami Kuvalayananda, Yoga helps cultivation of positive health through three integral steps:

1. Cultivation of correct psychological attitudes (maitri, karuna, mudita and upekshanam towards those who are sukha, duhkha, punya and apunya),
2. Reconditioning of neuro-muscular and neuro-glandular system – in fact, the whole body – enabling it to withstand stress and strain better,
3. Laying great emphasis on appropriate diet conducive to such a peak state of health, and encouraging the natural processes of elimination through various processes of nadi shuddhi or mala shuddhi.

To live a healthy life it is important to do healthy things and follow a healthy lifestyle. The modern world is facing a pandemic of lifestyle disorders that require changes to be made consciously by individuals themselves. Yoga places great importance on a proper and healthy lifestyle whose main components are:

1. Achar –Yoga stresses the importance of healthy activities such as exercise and recommends asana, pranayama and kriya on a regular basis. Cardio-respiratory health is one of the main by-products of such healthy activities.
2. Vichar –Right thoughts and right attitude towards life is vital for well being. A balanced state of mind is obtained by following the moral restraints and ethical observances (yama-niyama). As Mahatma Gandhi said, "there is enough in this world for everyone's need but not enough for any one person's greed".
3. Ahar – Yoga emphasises need for a healthy, nourishing diet that has an adequate intake of fresh water along with a well balanced intake of fresh food, green salads, sprouts, unrefined cereals and fresh fruits. It is important to be aware of the need for a satwica diet, prepared and served with love and affection.
4. Vihar – Proper recreational activities to relax body and mind are essential for good health. This includes proper relaxation, maintaining quietude of action-speech-thoughts and group activities wherein one loses the sense of individuality. Karma Yoga is an excellent method for losing the sense of individuality and gaining a sense of universality.

According to Yogacharini Meenakshi Devi Bhavanani, Director ICYER at Ananda Ashram in Pondicherry, Yoga has a step-by-step method for producing and maintaining perfect health at all levels of existence. She explains that social behaviour is first optimized through an understanding and control of the lower animal nature (pancha yama) and development and enhancement of the higher humane nature (pancha niyama). The body is then strengthened, disciplined, purified, sensitized, lightened, energized and made obedient to the higher will through asana. Universal pranic energy that flows through body-mind-emotions-spirit continuum is intensified and controlled through pranayama using breath control as a method to attain controlled expansion of the vital cosmic energy. The externally oriented senses are explored, refined, sharpened and made acute, until finally the individual can detach themselves from sensory impressions at will through pratyahara. The restless mind is then purified, cleansed, focused and strengthened through concentration (dharana). If these six steps are thoroughly understood and practiced then the seventh,

dhyana or meditation (a state of union of the mind with the object of contemplation) is possible. Intense meditation produces samadhi, or the enstatic feeling of Union, Oneness with the Universe. This is the perfect state of integration or harmonious health.

MODERN MEDICINE AND YOGA:
Though modern medicine may not share all of these concepts with Yoga, it is to be seen that there are a great many 'meeting points' for the construction of a healthy bridge between them. Both modern medicine and Yoga understand the need for total health and even the Word Health Organization has recently added a new dimension to the modern understanding of health by including spiritual health in its definition of the "state of health". Spiritual health is an important element of Yoga and now that even the WHO has come around to understanding this point of view, there is hope for a true unification of these two systems. Modern medicine has the ultimate aim and goal of producing a state of optimum physical and mental health thus ultimately leadings to the optimum well being of the individual. Yoga also aims at the attainment of mental and physical well being though the methodology does differ. While modern medicine has a lot to offer humankind in its treatment and management of acute illness, accidents and communicable diseases, Yoga has a lot to offer in terms of preventive, promotive and rehabilitative methods in addition to many management methods to tackle modern illnesses. While modern science looks outward for the cause of all ills, the Yogi searches the depth of his own self. This two way search can lead us to many answers for the troubles that plague modern man. The Shiva-Samhita lists the characters of a fully qualified disciple (shishya) as follows. "Endowed with great energy and enthusiasm, intelligent, heroic, learned in the scriptures, free from delusion…" Doesn't a true modern medical scientist require these very same qualities?

YOGA AND SOCIAL LIFE:
The science and art of Yoga, has for millennia guided man in his search for truth. Even in his personal and social life, Yoga has given him the tools and techniques with which he can find happiness, spiritual realization

and social harmony. Various Yogic concepts have guided man towards shaping his life and the interpersonal relationships in his social life. The Yogic concepts of samatvam (mental and emotional equanimity) and stitha prajna (the even minded, balanced human being) give us role models that we may strive to emulate.

An understanding of the pancha klesha (five psycho-physiological afflictions) and their role in the creation of stress and the stress response help us to know ourselves better and understand the how's and why's of what we do. The concept of the pancha kosha (the five layered existence of man as elucidated in the Taittiriya Upanishad) helps us to understand that we have more than only the physical existence and also gives us an insight into the role of the mind in causation of our physical problems as well as psychosomatic disorders. All of these concepts help us to look at life with a different perspective (yoga drishti) and strive to evolve consciously towards becoming Humane Beings. The concept of vairagya (dispassion or detachment) when understood and cultivated enables us to be dispassionate to the dwandwa (the pairs of opposites) such as praise-blame, hot-cold and the pleasant-unpleasant situations; that are part and parcel of our existence in this life.

The regular practice of Yoga as a 'Way of Life' (as defined by Yogamaharishi Dr Swami Gitananda Giri Guru Maharaj) helps us reduce the levels of physical, mental and emotional stress. This Yogic 'way of life' lays emphasis on right thought, right action, right reaction and right attitude. In short Pujya Swamiji defined Yogic living as "right-use-ness of body, emotions and mind".

The pancha yama and pancha niyama provide a strong moral and ethical foundation for our personal and social life. They guide our attitudes with regard to the right and wrong in our life and in relation to our self, our family unit and the entire social system. The yama-niyama provide a strong moral and ethical foundation for our personal and social life. They guide our attitudes with regard to the right and wrong in our life and in relation to our self, our family unit and the entire social system. These changes in our attitude and behaviour will go a long way in helping to prevent the very causes of stress in our life.

The pancha yama consisting of ahimsa (non – violence), satya (truthfulness), asteya (non-stealing), brahmacharya (proper channeling of creative impulse) and aparigraha (non – coveted-ness) are the "do not's" in a Yoga Sadhaka's life. Do not kill, do not be untruthful, do not steal, do not waste your god given creativity and do not covet that which does not belong to you. These guide us to say a big "NO" to our lower self and the lower impulses of violence etc. When we apply these to our life we can definitely have better personal and social relationships as social beings.

The pancha niyama consisting of saucha (cleanliness), santhosha (contentment), tapa (leading a disciplined life of austerity), svadhyaya (introspectional self analysis), and ishwara pranidhana (developing a sense of gratitude to the divine self) guide us with "DO'S" - do be clean, do be contented, do be disciplined, do self - study (introspection) and do be thankful to the divine for all of his blessings. They help us to say a big "YES" to our higher self and the higher impulses. Definitely a person with such qualities is a God-send to humanity. Even when we are unable to live the yama-niyama completely, even the attempt by us to do so will bear fruit and make each one of us a better person and help us to be of value to those around us and a valuable person to live with in our family and society. These are values which need to be introduced to the youth in order to make them aware and conscious of these wonderful concepts of daily living which are qualities to be imbibed with joy and not learnt with fear or compulsion.

Living a happy and healthy life on all planes is possible through the unified practice of Hatha Yoga especially when performed consciously and with awareness. Asana help to develop strength, flexibility, will power, good health, and stability and thus when practiced as a whole give a person a 'stable and unified strong personality'. Pranayama helps us to control our emotions which are linked to breathing and the pranamaya kosha (the vital energy sheath or body). Slow, deep and rhythmic breathing helps to control stress and overcome emotional hang-ups. The inner aspects of Yoga such as dharana and dhyana help us to focus our mid and dwell in it and thus help us to channel our creative energy in a wholistic manner towards the right type of evolutionary activities. They help us to understand our self better and in the process become better humans in this social world.

The adoption of Bhakti Yoga enables us to realise the greatness of the Divine and understand our puniness as compared to the power of the Divine or nature. We realize that we are but 'puppets on a string' following his commands on the stage of the world and then perform our activities with the intention of them being an offering to the divine and gratefully receive HIS/HER/ITS blessings.

DEVELOPING ESSENTIAL QUALITIES OF A GOOD HUMAN BEING

The universe is the Divine, nature is the Divine and every being is the Divine. You are the Divine and the Divine is you. Of course we must be careful that we don't go on an ego trip by misunderstanding this reality. The Divine is 'that' which is beyond name and form yet manifests to us through every name and form dear to us. He, She, It manifests to me personally through my father, my mother, my wife, my children, my students, my patients, my teachers, anyone and anything I choose to hold dear to my heart. Yoga is the dearest thing I hold to my heart and so for me the Divine is Yoga and Yoga is the Divine.

Patanjali says that the Divine, or iswara, is beyond the impurities of klesha (affliction or poison) and fructifications of the karma. He also implies in the Yoga Darshan that 'we' can become 'that' divinity itself when we rid ourselves of the impurities that prevent that awareness. Every yoganga, every part of Yoga, every part of life itself is a state of being, a state wherein we are a pure vehicle for the universal nature to manifest in its totality. The Divine is therefore for me a 'state of being'. If you are in that state, everything is Divine. On the other hand if we are not in such a state, then everything seems to be non-Divine.

Some of the important human qualities one must try and develop in the Yogic life are:
- Always be a good learner, ready to learn every moment
- Develop a strong self-introspective ability
- Be disciplined and dedicated towards the cause of Yoga
- Try to develop an understanding of the wholistic nature of Yoga physiology, philosophy and psychology along with a strong desire for spiritual evolution

- Be willing to learn from all situations
- Learn not to have an, "I know it all!" attitude.
- Develop a sense of empathy for others
- Be willing to sublimate our own EGO
- Have a good sense of humour and laugh at yourself without reservation
- Try to motivate others by self-example and lead the way as a true acharya.
- Always have devotion to the guru who has guided you for guru droha or treachery to one's guru is considered the worst sin.
- Do your best and leave the rest for everything happens only for our spiritual evolution.

CONCLUSION:
Love for Yoga is the key component of a Yoga life. Of course, joy and fun are part of the Yoga life at all times. Develop an ardent desire to evolve on the path towards oneness and keep working on it non stop. Compassion, empathy and love are important dynamics that are to be worked on while petty egocentric stuff needs to be kept at the bottom of the pile. The ability to sublimate one's individuality for the sake of the group is an important part of the Yoga life. Constant growth through satsangha is very useful, and being open to correction and change at all times is a must. We need to remember that the guru is not just the physical manifestation but is a spirit of guidance that can manifest through so many vehicles. One must be constant on the lookout for its manifestation as such a spirit may manifest through our partner, our children, our neighbours, our students, our friends and often through our worst enemies too. I have found that people who consider me their worst enemy have actually helped my growth more than some who have always been caring and considerate. The ones who always looking for chances to degrade me keep me on my toes, and make me do the best I can without fail. They are the stimulant that enables the best to flower through me. When they play such a great role in my life, is not it right that I thank them for being a manifestation of the guru spirit too? Yoga is not just performing some contortionist poses or huffing and puffing some pranayama or sleeping our way through any so-called meditation. It is an integrated way of life in which awareness and

consciousness play a great part in guiding our spiritual evolution through life in the social system itself and not in some remote cave in the mountains or hut in the forest. As my beloved Guru-Father Pujya Swamiji Gitananda Giri Guru Maharaj said "Yoga is the science and art of right-useness of body, emotions and mind".

Through the dedicated practice of Yoga as a way of life, we can become a truly balanced humane being (sthita prajna) with the following qualities as described in the Bhagavad Gita:
- Beyond passion, fear and anger. (II.56)
- Devoid of possessiveness and egoism. (II.71)
- Firm in understanding and un-bewildered. (V.20)
- Engaged in doing good to all beings. (V.25)
- Friendly and compassionate to all. (XII.13)
- Having no expectation, pure and skilful in action. (XII.16)

The Yogi wishes peace and happiness not only for himself, but also for all beings on all the different planes of existence. He is not an "individualist" seeking salvation for only himself but on the contrary is an "universalist" seeking to live life in the proper evolutionary manner to the best of his ability and with care and concern for his human brethren as well as all beings on all planes of existence.

"Om, loka samasta sukhino bhavanthu sarve janaha sukhino bhavanthu"
"Om shanti, shanti, shanti Om"

CLAIMING ONE'S BIRTHRIGHT THROUGH YOGA
Ammaji, Yogacharini Meenakshi Devi Bhavanani
Director and Ashram Acharya,
ICYER at Ananda Ashram, Pondicherry.
www.icyer.com

"Health and happiness are your birthright! Claim them!" thundered the "Lion of Modern Yoga" Yogamaharishi Dr. Swami Gitananda Giri Guru Maharaj. "You are born to be healthy and happy. But, the goal of life is Moksha – Freedom!"

We live in "Topsy – Turvy Times", when ancient values have been flipped onto their heads. One rarely meets a truly "healthy" or "happy" person. In fact, for the vast majority of the human race, health and happiness are distant dreams. Illness, depression, conflict, sorrow, stress, tension and frustration are the "birthright" even of young children in modern times. Billions of dollars are expended by the health industry. Medical science can put pig valves into human hearts and transplant vital organs. Super Specialty Hospitals abound. The pharmaceutical industry produces a huge amount of life-saving drugs. Why, then, is a truly healthy, happy person such a rarity?

Modern man, like the Biblical Essau, has sold his birthright for a "mess of porridge". Like Judas, he has betrayed his Christ Consciousness, his Cosmic Consciousness, for less than "30 pieces of silver".

Swami Gitananda has put before us a simple reason for this sad state of affairs. He advised. "If you want to be healthy, do healthy things. If you want to be happy, do happy things." People cry, "I want to be healthy." Then, they indulge in bad habits like tobacco and alcohol, spend late-hours watching television, do not exercise properly, and do not drink enough water. Others moan, "I want to be happy!" but they fight, they gossip, they quarrel, they criticize, they delight in conflict, in violence, in defeating others, and crushing competition under their feet. It is irrational to expect that by doing unhealthy things, one can be healthy. It is irrational to believe that by doing unhappy things, one can be happy. Yes, man is an irrational animal indeed!

Yoga is the ancient science of India which shows man not only how to claim his birthright of health and happiness, but also how to obtain the goal of life – Moksha. Any scientist worth his salt begins his career by studying the laws of nature and the basic theorems and tenets of his science. The Yogic scientist is no exception to this rule. The physicist studies the physical laws of nature – gravity, momentum etc, the chemist studies the chemical properties of matter, the biologist studies life forms, and the doctors, the anatomy of the human body. This is the "field" within which they will work, observing the laws of action and reaction, the laws of cause – effect relationship, within that limited spectrum.

For the Yogi, the entire Universe and everything in it is his "field of research." He studies the Universal Laws, which operate within this field. The Law of Karma, the Law of Cause – Effect, is an important Law for him. The Yogi knows that the Laws which govern the microcosm also govern the macrocosm, and so, he understands that by studying himself, his "small self," his "own self", his own body, mind and emotions, he can understand the "Big Self", the Atman, Brahman, This process in Yoga is called "Swadhyaya" or "Self Study" and it is the fourth Niyama of Patanjali's Ashtanga Yoga. The Rishis, Cosmic Scientists, have taught, "Without moving out of one's own cave, one can comprehend the mighty Universe." They realised that Universal Truths lay within one's very own heart. "Man, know thyself" is the admonition which was written on the entrance to the Greek Temple at Delphi. This is the starting point of all endeavours. This is the starting point in the long journey to claim one's birthright. Alexander Pope, the great 18th century English poet, wrote, "Man, know thy self / Presume not God to scan / The proper study of Mankind / is man."

Through this "Self Study" the Yogi discovers that human nature is governed by an inexorable Law – and the very Law which governs his nature – is the very Law which governs the Universe. This Law is called "Sanathana Dharma" or "The Eternal Law" – This Law is unbreakable. One has no choice but to discover it, and then, live in harmony with that Eternal Law. Only then will one be entitled to enjoy one's birthright – health and happiness. The Christian Bible teaches, "The wages of sin is death." "Sin" is nothing more than defiance, rebellion and disobedience

to the Eternal Law. Yogamaharishi Dr. Swami Gitananda Giri taught his students: "You cannot break The Law. You can only break yourself over The Law." How do we know if we are "breaking the Law"? The results are there for all to see: sickness, suffering, unhappiness, conflict, stress, and tension.

One might retort – "But I am unhealthy! I am unhappy! I am not breaking Law! I am not an outlaw!" Look again! Indeed, such a person must be breaking the Law, whether knowingly or unknowingly. Remember! Even in human jurisprudence, "Ignorance of the Law is no excuse." No court on earth will excuse a law – breaker who pleads "ignorance of the law". All citizens are expected to not only know the Law, but also, to abide by it, so that the society may flourish in a harmonious manner. But, who wants to be unhealthy? Who wants to be unhappy? If these are the result of breaking Natural Law, then why do people do it? The answer is pure and simple: Ignorance. The Sanskrit word for "ignorance" is "Avidya". Maharishi Patanjali, the sage who codified the principles of Yoga 2500 years ago in 196 magnificently concise Sutras, calls "Avidya" or "Ignorance" as the "Mother Klesha". A Klesha is a hindrance, an obstacle to spiritual growth. Basically, Kleshas are the root cause of all human problems. There are the Pancha Klesha or "Five Hindrances". Sometimes "Klesha" is translated as "A Knot of the Heart". It prevents the human being from further spiritual advancement and drags the human into the mire of misery. The other four Kleshas are Asmita (egoism, the sense of separation, the sense of I), Raga (attraction, pleasure), Dwesha (aversion and pain) and Abinivesha (clinging to life, the survival instinct). These are the "obstacles", which stand between man and his desire to claim his birthright of health and happiness. But, the root of all obstacles is Avidya – ignorance - ignorance of the Law, and hence, the constant attempt to "break the Law."

What is ignorance? Look at the word. It is composed mostly of the word "ignore". "Ignore" implies "a refusal to see". If we "ignore" someone, it implies a deliberate attempt to cut this person out of the field of our awareness. If we attend a gathering and find someone we have aversion towards (Dwesha) present, we usually "ignore" him or her, literally, turning "our back on him or her" so that we do not have to "see him or her" or "acknowledge him or her."

But, if ignorance of the Universal Law causes us to break The Law, and hence, results in disease and unhappiness, why do we as humans continue on this path to death and destruction? Because we are taught, and we willingly accept this falsehood, that we are not responsible for our own health and happiness. We have given over the responsibility for our own health to the doctor, and have asked him to find us a pill, or cut something out of our body, or stick something into it, and make us healthy again. We have given the responsibility of our happiness to the government, the society, to the media, to the entertainment industry, to anti-depressant medicines - and ask them to "please us, to give us what we want, to make us happy."

We have sold the most precious quality we possess as humans – "Manas" or conscious awareness – and its twin virtues, independence and self – initiative to the various powerful lobbies, which govern our lives. And, they turn, most benevolently "put us to sleep", sedate us, put us under anesthesia, so we no longer feel the pain inherent in breaking The Law. We are hypnotized into a fitful sleep from our childhood to our old age, and into the funeral pyre itself. We are lulled into a somnolent state in order to make our life's journey bearable, with a minimum of pain – we are neither healthy nor happy, but blissfully numb and anesthetized.

Why should our entire social, political, educational, business, commercial, media, entertainment structure be geared to keeping us numb and dumb? For a simple reason – there's plenty of money and power in unhappiness and disease. But, there's no money in health and happiness. How would doctors and the huge drug industry support themselves if all were healthy? Would we watch mindless violence and sex and vulgarity in cinemas and television if we were truly happy? Would the manufacturers of weapons of mass destruction flourish financially if all were happy and healthy? It is beneficial to all the world's commercial interests that the five billion people on the planet are kept sick and unhappy, in a state of unfulfilled desire and thus, in constant frustration.

As an example close to home, look at the field of dentistry. When I came to Pondy in 1968, there was one dentist in town. I did not know anyone who had problems with their teeth. Cavities were rare. On the contrary,

I was struck by the beautiful, white healthy teeth of our Indian people. Even villagers had dazzling smiles! Life was simple. Processed foods were a luxury. Natural food was the norm.

Cut to the present scenario. The number of dentists in Pondicherry numbers more than 500! Children as young as four years of age have cavities and dental problems. I don't have to tell you professionals where the problem lies. It is obvious! The abundance of refined foods, sugars, sweets, soft drinks, ice creams, lack of oral hygiene have destroyed the nation's teeth! The good old neem stick has been discarded as "old fashioned" and we now spend Rs.20 on a toothbrush and Rs.50 on toothpaste, which is not one-hundredth as effective as the old neem twig! Is this progress? Is this obedience to Natural Law? Is this health? Is this happiness? The villager cannot afford to buy toothbrush and toothpaste – this would cost him one day's wages – this "progress" has not only taken his health, but also his happiness. He will "become unhappy "because he does not have the money to buy such items!" Should not the emphasis in social dentistry be on spreading awareness of the horrendous damage caused to the teeth by these modern junk foods and drink? But, emphasis seems to be more focused on cure, rather than prevention. Lip service is given to these ideas but the powerful commercial lobbies are quick to squelch any effective activism on these subjects. This is not only in the field of dentistry. It is the fact in every single aspect of life. There is no money or glory or power in prevention, but plenty of it in cure! Instead of educating people to "obey Natural Law", the modern trend is to repair people who have "broken themselves over that Law."

Avidya, ignorance! It is a disease, which is more deadly than an atomic bomb. It has already burst upon the earth and is enveloping all mankind in its black, poisonous mushroom cloud. It is the root cause of all unhappiness and disease.

"Vidya" – wisdom, knowledge – is the opposite of "Avidya" or ignorance. It basically means, "to see". The Rishis were "men who saw Reality as it is." If we wish to claim our birthright of health and happiness, we must "arise and awake." We must open our eyes to see and our ears to hear. When this "awakening" occurs, one will be drawn to the Yogic science. It is the start of the long spiritual journey.

The "core concept" in accepting Yoga as a way of life is embedded in the word "Responsibility." One must be prepared to accept "total responsibility" for one's own life, total responsibility for one's thoughts, words and deeds, total responsibility for one's own health and happiness. This is, in essence, obedience to the "Eternal Law" which states, "All Karma – all action – has its reaction – and that re-action will always rebound on the one who committed the action." Just as the Sudarshan (discus) of Lord Vishnu followed the sage Durvasa wherever he ran as he tried to hide, until he made amends to King Ambarishi for harming him, so also the "reaction" of our "action" will follow us wherever we go, until we "pay out" the Karma in consciousness. In short, if we do unhappy things, we will be unhappy. If we do unhealthy things, we will be unhealthy. There is no "breaking" this Law and even the best doctor, the best dentist, the best entertainer cannot keep our Karma forever at bay. The sign on the Yogi's door (whether the door leads to his palace or the door leads to his cave) reads. "The buck stops here." That is, the Yogi takes total and complete responsibility for himself and everything which happens him and makes a conscious choice to "live within the Law", rather than choosing to be an "out law."

The word "responsibility" also has another aspect. Broken into two parts it reads "respond – ability", or "the ability to respond". The Yogic way of life cultivates and values consciousness and awareness. Hence the Yogi develops the "ability to respond" correctly to any given situation. The correct "response" will produce a "positive effect" and the result of such a positive action – choice is overall health, harmony and happiness.

Yoga is the Science of Consciousness, becoming aware of Universal Laws and obeying those Laws in thought, word and deed. Obedience to the Law produces health and happiness. Disobedience produces disease and suffering. As a scientist, the Yogi employs all the tools of any great science: he possesses an elaborate terminology which helps him define and understand the problem; he possesses equipment and tools for his research – Asanas, Pranayama, Concentration Practices, Mantras, Cleansing techniques etc.

He / she enjoys access to a great body of theoretical concepts, accumulated through hundreds of generations of "spiritual experiments"

conducted by the great Rishis who have preceded him. This "theory" is recorded in the Vedas, the Upanishads, the Bhagavad Gita, the Yoga Sutras, the Gheranda Samhita, the Hatha Yoga Pradipika and other ancient scriptures. His laboratory, his field of research, is his own body, emotions and mind and his relationship and correspondence to the Universe. The Yogi is a detached observer who carefully records his data and comes to his own conclusions based on his own direct observation and experiences.

He begins with this primary hypothesis – the Universe is Cosmos, it is not Chaos. "Cosmos" implies "Order", and "Order" Implies "Laws". He sets out to discover those Laws and to observe the working of those Laws in his own life and in the lives of others. The Yogi then attempts to "apply" his findings in a practical manner – in his own life, coming to the same "realisations" as those enjoyed by the Rishis of old. Health and happiness manifest automatically in such a life, which attunes itself to Cosmic Law. Health and happiness are automatic by – products when Avidya or ignorance is dispelled and Vidya – seeing reality for what it is – develops. The Yogi follows the "Great Law of Virtue" which is elaborated in the Yogic tradition as the Yamas or Moral Restraints and the Niyamas, the Ethical Observances. The Maha Vratas, the Mighty Vows of Virtue, which the Yamas and Niyamas are sometimes called, reflect the Sanathana Dharma or the Eternal Law. The Yogi develops a love for virtue, a love for the Law. He realises "Virtue is its own reward." He attunes his own microcosm to the rhythm of the macrocosm. He moves with Nature, not against it. Nature is his friend, with whom he lives in harmony, and not an enemy to be conquered or exploited.

"Sanathana Dharma" is difficult to translate. It can be called "The Eternal Law", "The Cosmic Law", even "The Structure of the Universe As It Is". "Sanathana" means "eternal" – That which was, which is, and which shall always be – unchanging, self-created, unborn, undying. "Dharma" takes its root meaning from "Dhar" which means "stability, even-ness, balance." The English word "durable" has come from "Dhar" – "that which endures. "Dharma" is hence that which gives stability. Stability is an essential component of health. As any good doctor knows, the best news he can give anxious relatives is that the patient has "stabilized." Stability is also an essential component of happiness. Nothing creates

more misery than an unstable family, unstable romantic relationships, unstable work or social environments. Sanathana Dharma sometimes is more loosely defined as "The Law of Virtue". Virtue creates stability. Clean, pure, restrained, controlled, conscious aware living is the basis of all virtue. Such qualities create personal, interpersonal and intrapersonal stability. Hence, one becomes aware of the necessity of obeying "The Law of Virtue", if one wishes to be qualified to claim one's birthright as health and happiness. As Yogamaharishi Dr. Swami Gitananda put it so succinctly – "Following Yama – Niyama, obeying The Cosmic Law, is "No-option Yoga" for those who wish to spiritually evolve themselves in health and happiness.

Our ancients linked particular diseases to certain lapses in character. These linkages can be found in many Puranas. Arthritis is linked to greed, refusal to let go, or to share. Digestive problems were linked to hoarding, excessive, selfish accumulation. The old idea that diseases were caused by a moral lapse had much truth. Interestingly enough, modern medicine is also coming to a similar conclusion, though by a different route. Research findings have enabled medical men to draw up "personality profiles" for cancer patients, heart attack patients, diabetics, AIDS patients and so on. Character creates circumstances. Character is composed mostly of the word "act". The manner in which we habitually "act" forms our "character." Our actions determine whether we are healthy or unhealthy, happy or unhappy. This is the essence of Sanathana Dharma. We create our own destiny by our thoughts, our words and our actions. There is no such thing as an "innocent victim" in the Universal Scheme of Things.

The Yogi grows in consciousness and spirit till he becomes an "Adhikarin" a "Fit Person" for "Realising Reality". He becomes competent to "claim his birthright of health and happiness." But, that is only the beginning of his journey. He has arisen! He has been awakened! And now it is his duty to "stop not till the goal of Moksha" is reached. But, though the pilgrimage is long and arduous, the Universe (Herself / Himself / Itself) grants him his birthright – health and happiness as the reward for obeying Natural Law. He has the health, strength and good cheer to make his Cosmic Journey and he has the happiness to enjoy his travels in space and consciousness. Buoyed by this spiritual legacy, the Yogi now has a raft

to cross the ocean of Samskara. "Avidya" – ignorance of Universal Law – is banished by "Vidya", the Light of Conscious Awareness. His eyes are opened. He sees! He sees! He sees! Happily and healthily he realizes that he lives not on a small planet, in a small galaxy, tiny as a grain of sand. He is a Universal Being, a Universal Citizen obeying the Laws of the Cosmos. And the Universe is his own, his native land!

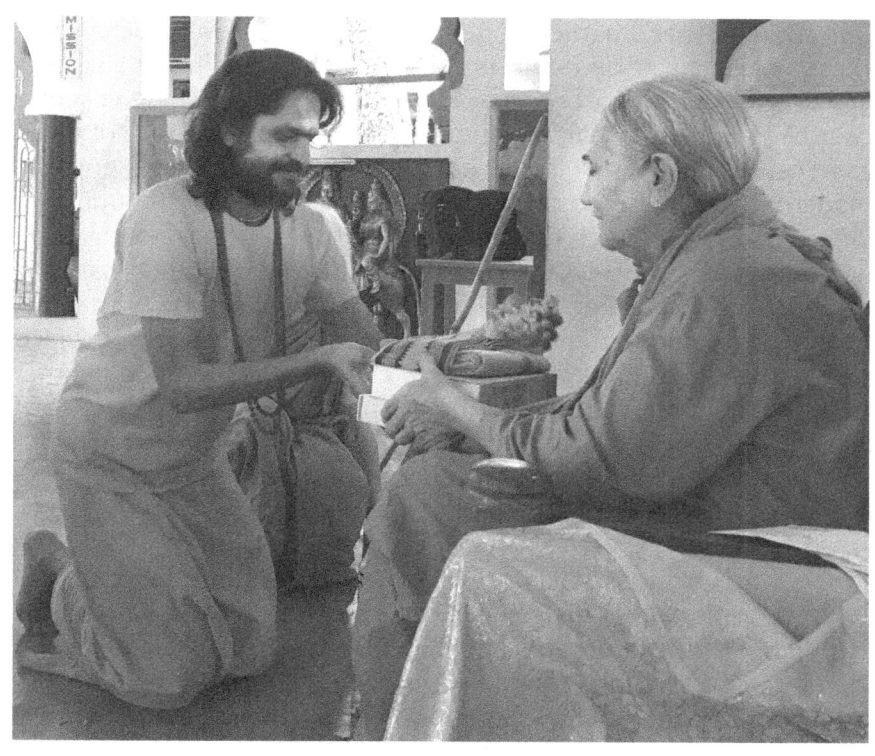

Yogachariya Jnandev with his Guru Ammaji Yogacharini Meenakshi Devi Bhavanani at Kambali Swami Temple, Puducherry

AMMAJI, YOGACHARINI MEENAKSHI DEVI BHAVANANI

Yogacharini Meenakshi Devi Bhavanani popularly known worldwide as Ammaji, is Director and Resident Acharya of the world famous International Centre for Yoga Education and Research (ICYER at Ananda Ashram) and Yoganjali Natyalayam at Pondicherry. She is the Dharmapatni and senior most disciple of the internationally acclaimed Yoga master, Yogamaharishi Dr. Swami GitanandaGiri Guru Maharaj and has devoted her life to his teachings and to institutions founded by him. She is a prolific author with 12 books, including two books of poetry to her credit. She is Editor of Satya Press and her defining books on "The History of Yoga from Ancient to Modern Times- Part 1 &2" are path breaking effort hailed as the "Defining publications on the history of Yoga to date." Her book, "The Rishis and Rakshashas" traces the transformational aspects in India over the past five decades. She has trained many thousands of students in Yoga and Bharatanatyam in the past five decades and is considered a pioneer in bringing the Performing Fine Arts and Yoga to the common people in Pondicherry.

She has been recipient of many National and State Awards such as "Yogamani" in 1986 from the President of India Shri Zail Singh Ji and "Bhaskar Award" by Bharat Nirman as one of 50 eminent Indians honoured during the 50th year of Indian Independence for their contribution to Indian culture and spirituality. In 1999 she was given the "PuduvaiKalaimamani" Award for her work in BharataNatyam by the Pondicherry Government.

She is presently a Member of the National Board for Yoga and Naturopathy in the Ministry of AYUSH, Govt of India. In the past she has served on the Pondicherry University Academic Council, the Central Council for Research in Yoga & Naturopathy as well as the Morarji Desai National Institute of Yoga under Ministry of Health, Government of India. Ammaji is considered one of the major International leaders of the modern Yoga movement. Though born in the USA in 1943, she came to India in 1967 and has lived here ever since. She was awarded Indian Citizenship on November 30th, 1992, in her own words "the proudest day of my life."

What is the traditional meaning of Yoga?

Word Yoga comes from ancient Indian Language Sanskrita which means adding or joining. Yoga means adding or joining individual self with higher self. Yoga is process, path, and goal. We are living our lives and busy in doing one or other things. Yoga is the transformation of our attitude from the doing to being. Yoga is mindful or conscious living where we become aware and take responsibility for every choice we make.

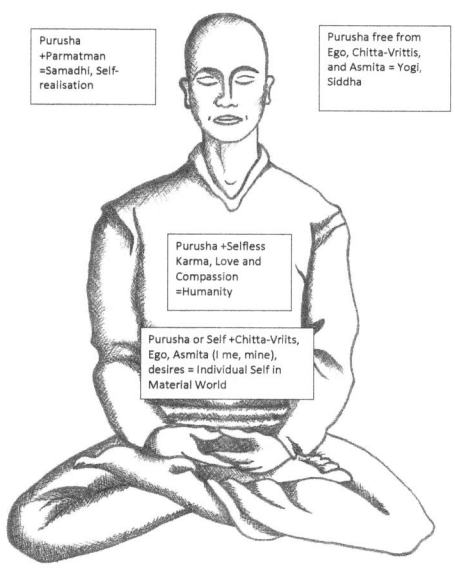

Why should one Practice Yoga?

Everyone has their own goals or aims to practice yoga. Many practice yoga for its physical benefits to improve flexibility, strength and general health and well being. Many also practice yoga for mental peace and well being. While a wide range of group follows yoga as a therapy. There are still many yoga Sadhakas following yoga as a path to self-realisation.

Is yoga goal or a path?

Yoga is goal or end in the form of attaining Samadhi, Moksha, Liberation or self-realisation. Yoga is also the path and provides us all the tools, practices, kriyas and prakriyas which helps us to achieve the goal to Samadhi or perfection. Yoga also has all the scientific physical, psychological, and spiritual concepts and ideas on how to free ourselves from ego and attachment causing pain and suffering.

Where is the Origin of Yoga?

Yoga is one of the most beautiful and practical path, approach or lifestyle given to humanity by Sanatana dharma or Hindu culture from Indian subcontinent known as Bharata or India now. It was known as Hindustan or Bharatavarsha before the partition in 1947.

What is Hinduism?

Hindu belief system is based on "The idea that each human life has the potential to attain self-realisation". This idea goes further deeper that in one or other life we will find our way to liberation. Hinduism is also a lifestyle based on very scientific concepts and principals to fulfil our Dharma and duties in various stages of life known as Chatur Ashrams. Every practice, rituals and ceremonies are detailed in Vedas, Upanishads, etc.

What are Chatur Dharmas or Ashrams?

Hinduism or Vedic culture divides life into four phases, detailing how to live our life to find our real potentiality in each of the stages.

1. Brahmacharya- Ashram this from birth to 25 years where our energy,

time and effort should be to learn, practice and master all the life skills to fulfil our Dharma we are meant to achieve in this lifetime.
2. Grihastha Ashram- In this phase we enter into the household where we make a family, fulfil all the material needs of our family and society to your best.
3. Sanyasa Ashram- In this phase from 50 to 75 years we renounce from Grahistha and take responsibility to help younger generations as educators or guides by sharing our life experiences and skills.
4. Vanaprastha Ashram- 75 years onward we renounce entirely and move from social life into solitude to devote life to self-realisation or Samadhi.

What are Chatura Yugas?

Hinduism and Samkhya classify time or ages in four phases- 1. Satayuga, 2. Treta Yuga, 3. Dwapara Yuga and 4. Kaliyuga. Four yugas make one Kalpa or one cycle or Brahma or universe to go through the period from beginning to the end. Through these four cycle Prana (subtle electromagnetic eternal force), Akasha (ether or voidness) and Parmatman or Supreme consciousness are transforming into various evolutes to manifest everything in the whole universe.

What are Vedas?

Vedas are four sacred Hindu scriptures written in Sanskrita from Self-realised Yogis or Rishis to help every human being to attain Samadhi or perfection. Veda is derived from root 'Vid' means to know. Veda means knowledge.

Modern historians say that Vedas were written between 5000 to 6000 years ago, but Vedas or Vedic expertise is much older as this is a period where evidence of the written Vedas was found.

Vedas from the ancient time where taught Guru-Shisya Paramaparai,

the teacher will pass knowledge to his or her disciple orally. The teaching of Vedas are still efficient and useful, and hence the dating is not important.

What are four Vedas?

The Rig-Veda – This is first and oldest of Vedas written in praise of various forms of divine and gods. Rig means ritual, and it contains mainly hymns and prayers (Mantras) in the worship of the universal or divine forces known as Devas and Devis

The Yajur Veda- Yajur means ceremony, and it mainly describes how to perform the rituals or Yajnas. This Veda also explains how to perform various rites and rituals at different phases of life at the time of birth, marriage, Sannyasa, death, etc.

Sama-Veda is third Veda detailing chants, melodies and correct methods to sing during yajna ceremonies. Sama means singing; the scriptures of these categories contain many other mantras as well as strict rules how to chant these mantras according to mystic vibrations.

Atharva-Veda -Atharva means a priest who knows the secret lore; these scriptures describe many different kinds of worship and invocations. In a broader sense, many other scriptures on knowledge about material aspects of life are also counted in the Atharva, like the Ayurveda.

Is Yoga part of Hinduism?

Yes, Yoga has its roots and origins in Hinduism. Yoga is the compilation of all the practices, kriyas and prakriyas of Hindu lifestyle leading any human being to attain Self-realisation. To understand Yoga in its real sense and holistic meanings we have to study and follow many Hindu scriptures like Bhagavata Gita, Yoga-Upanishads, Yoga-Chudamani, Vijnana Bhairava Tantra along with Yoga Sutras.

Do I Have to be a Hindu to Practice Yoga?

No, Yoga in its true meaning is the union of self with higher self. In Samkhya Yoga explains the concept of Purusha (Individual Self) and Parmatman (higher self). Samadhi or Self-realisation is the union of Individual Self with higher Self. Through the practice of yoga, you are aspiring to become a better human being and choose to live your life consciously on the evolutionary path. So yoga will make you a better Hindu, Muslim, Christian, etc.

How does yoga evolve through various ages from Satayuga to Kaliyuga?

Lord Shiva, the Adiyogi or first yogi, shared yoga with his wife Shakti or Parvati and then with the Sapta Rishis, seven sages, who then created seven primary schools of yoga. These schools disseminated into hundreds of forms of yoga.

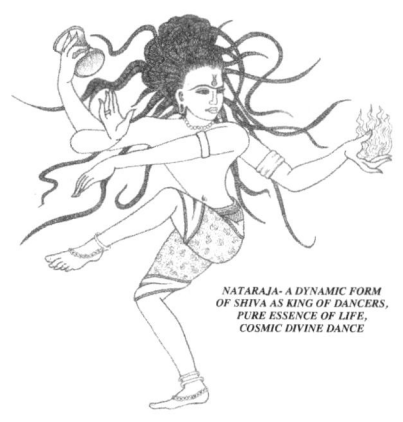

NATARAJA- A DYNAMIC FORM OF SHIVA AS KING OF DANCERS, PURE ESSENCE OF LIFE, COSMIC DIVINE DANCE

From then Yoga in ancient time flourished across Indian continent, known as Bharat-varsh. We have Yoga Vashishtha (dialogue between Lord Rama and Sage Vasishtha) explaining many paths of yoga to attain liberation in many beautiful stories of great yogis and yoginis. Then we have Bhagavata Gita (dialogue between Arjuna and Lord Krishna) just before the biggest battle of Mahabharata. Later we have Vijnana Bhairava Tantra and Shiva Samhita detailing a much easier and accessible path of yoga through many meditative, contemplative and kundalini yoga practices.

More recently we had Hatha Yoga Pradipika and Gheranda Samhita

detailing purifying practices, asana, mudra, pranayama and some concentration techniques.

What is Raja Yoga?

Raja means Royal or Supreme, while Yoga means Union or Samadhi. Raja Yoga is step by step approach or path for any individual to follow to reach self-realisation. Raja Yoga is also known as Ashtanga Yoga or Yoga of Eight Limbs. Maharishi Patanjali in Yoga Sutras details every aspect of human mind, its nature and how attain purity and stillness of mind to transcend our awareness to experience higher or divine self.

Raja Yoga begins with a very strong foundation Yamas and Niyamas, followed by Asana, Pranayama, Pratyahara, Dharana, Dhyana and Samadhi. Lord Krishna in Bhagavad Gita mentions Raja Yoga as the highest path for Yogis who are seeking enlightenment. First four limbs are known as Bahiranga Yoga, and other four are classified as Antaranga Yoga.

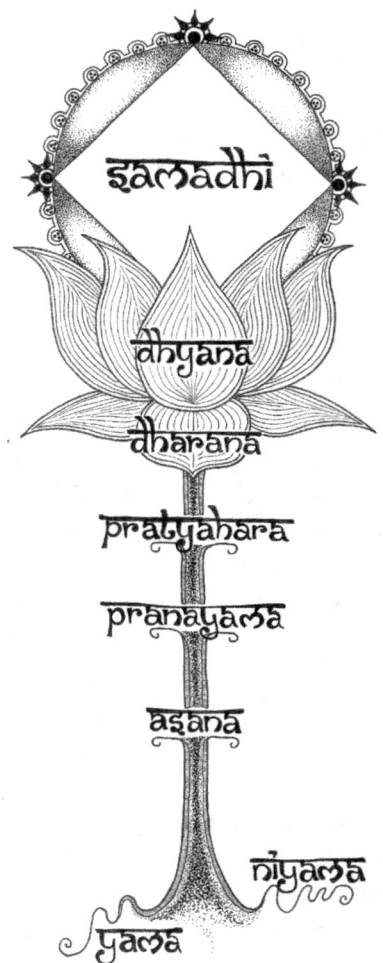

What is Bahiranga and Antaranga Yoga?

Ashtanga or Raja is divided into two parts, Bahiranga and Antaranga. Bahira means outer or physical, and Anga implies to limb or part. First, four limbs of yoga- Yamas, Niyamas, Asana and Pranayama are known as Bahiranga or physical, external evolutionary practices to prepare for Antaranga Yoga.

Antar means Inner, and Anga implies to Limb or part. Antaranga Yoga is advanced internal and more profound aspect of yoga at the deeper subconscious and unconscious levels through Pratyahara, Dharana, Dhyana and Samadhi.

What are Eight Limbs of Raja Yoga?

1. Yama (restrains)
2. Niyama (observances)
3. Asana (posture, pose or seat)
4. Pranayama (subtle energy work)
5. Pratyahara (sensory withdrawal)
6. Dharana (concentration)
7. Dhyana (meditation)
8. Samadhi (Union or self-realisation)

What is Hatha Yoga?

Hatha means forceful or vigorous. The Sanskrita word Hatha is composed of two syllables: ha and tha. Ha stands for the seer, the Self, the soul (Purusa), and for the sun (Surya) and the in breath (prana). Tha represents nature (Prakriti), consciousness {citta), the moon (Chandra) and the outbreak (Apana). Yoga, as already noted, means union. Hatha yoga, therefore, means the union of Purusa with Prakriti, consciousness with the soul, the sun with the moon, and prana with Apana.

Hatha Yoga is branch or Yoga detailing the practices to purify our body and mind through Shat-Karmas, followed with balancing the right-left, solar-lunar, prana-Apana, masculine-feminine energies. This path further leads us to master our senses and mind leading to Dharana or concentration practices. Hatha Yoga Pradipika and Gheranda Samhita are key Hatha Yoga scriptures.

What is Karma Yoga?

Karma means action, or deeds we do. Karma includes all our thoughts and feelings, words and speech and physical activities. Karma is also what we do ourselves, encourage or discourage or pay someone else to do.

In Bhagavata Gita Lord Krishna explains the importance of Niskama Karma, means selfless or desireless action. Karma Yoga is doing or fulfilling all our Dharma or duties free from any expectations or fruits. Krishan says- "do your best and leave the rest". Karma Yoga is service to human life and humanity. Every action at the level of thoughts, feelings, emotions and physical activities are devoted to the divine cause.

What is Mantra Yoga?

A mantra is a sacred word, syllable, sound or phrase in Ancient language Sanskrit. Each Mantra has its physical, psychological, energetic and spiritual power. 'Manah' means mind and 'Tra' means tool. The mantra is a tool of mind to focus and enhance its abilities.

Mantra yoga uses chanting and repetition with focus on their meaning to lead our mind from distracted states to higher focused states. This leads Sadhaka to transcend their mind from lower planes of mind to higher planes of mind. Yogis explain that by chanting the mantras, you are creating specific vibrations to evoke various divine energies leading to higher states of consciousness in meditation.

What is Tantra Yoga?

Word 'tan' means body and 'tra' means tool. Tantra uses the body as a tool evolve from lower to higher states of consciousness. It explains two aspects of energies regarding Shiva-Shakti, Prana-Apana, Right-Left, or Male-Female. It uses shat-karmas to purify the body to prepare for the evolutionary spiritual journey. Tantra details many asanas, kriyas, pranayama, mudras, and jnana yoga kriyas or visualisations balance our energies and gradually attain perfect balance or union of these two polar energies within our own body. Here our energy and mind will naturally flow inward and find their union back to the source where they originated.

What is Jnana Yoga?

Jnana (wisdom or knowledge) is known to be the most advanced of all the paths of Yoga, requiring strong will, determination and intellect. In Jnana yoga, the mind or consciousness is used to seek the truth or reality through introspection or enquiry into its true nature.

Through positive contemplations on spiritual principals and nature of Purusha (soul) and Paramatma (supreme soul), one frees the Self from ego and its attachment with worldly desires. Once the self is free from Maya or illusion, it attains Samadhi or Union with Higher or Universal-Self. This is achieved by regularity, and repetition of these mental techniques of self-enquiry. Jnana Yoga describes four pillars of Knowledge or Jnana.

Viveka- is discrimination or intelligence which helps us to be aware, know and differentiate between the real and unreal, the permanent and the temporary, and the self and that which is not.

Vairagya- is detachment from all the worldly and mundane desires possessions.

Shad-Sampati -consists of 6 values or principals to master our mind and emotions.

Mumukshutva- Mumukshutva is an intense passion for liberation

What is Dhyana Yoga?

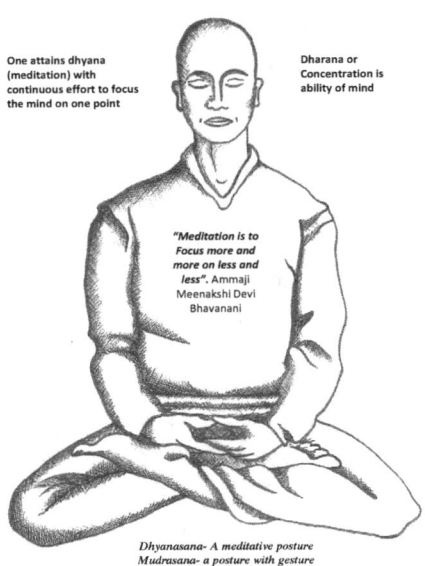

Dhyanasana- A meditative posture
Mudrasana- a posture with gesture

Dhyana means meditation or one-pointed concentration. Dhyana Yoga uses various tools or techniques known as Jnana Yoga Kriyas or Dharana to focus the mind on one point. Using meditation one gradually liberates the mind from its attachment with pain, suffering and whirlpools caused due to desires, ego and Asmita.

Dhyana Yogis use techniques which can be external or internal like focussing our mind on a mandala or shape, breath, chakras, or internal energy flows, or a point.

What is Kriya Yoga?

Patanjali describes Tapas- austerity or disciplined practice, Swadhyaya – self-study or introspection, and Iswara Pranidhanani – devotion or faith in the divine cause. Kriya Yoga outlines the path of subtle yogic kriyas or exercises to be practised mindfully, with inner reflection and love in the divine.

Yogananda Paramahamsa took Kriya Yoga to the west and taught this path of yoga to the broader community. Before him, it was a secret path of yoga only for spiritual seekers.

What is Pranayama Yoga?

Prana is the subtlest form of vital cosmic energy. Prana means most delicate energy which can not be broken further. This Prana is eternal energy which exists before, during and at the end of creation.

Pranayama is enhancing this energy which allows us to experience vibrations of prana. Prana or energy transforms from one to another form from material to non-material, kinetic to potential. In Pranayama

Yoga a Sadhaka aims to control, refine, and enhance these subtle energies and transcends them to flow back into their source where they originated. This leads to the natural awakening of our true potentiality and Samadhi.

What is Kundalini Yoga?

Kundalini is an ancient path of yogic science or path of transformation, expansion and enhancement of consciousness through the awakening of Kundalini or Serpent power. Once awakened the Sadhaka guides this energy through Chakras leading to the Sahashrara or crown

centre. This includes bringing union or Prana or Shiva into Apana or Shakti employing Hatha Yoga Kriyas, Pranayama, Bandhas, Mudras and Mantras. Kundalini Yoga is the balanced path between Kriya, Bhakti, Hatha, Mantra, Jnana and Raja Yoga.

What are the Seven Chakras?

1. Mooladhara Chakra (Root Chakra)
2. Swadhisthana Chakra (Self-dwelling or Pelvic centre)
3. Manipura Chakra (Jewel or Solar Plexus)
4. Anahata Chakra (Unstruck or heart centre)
5. Vishuddha Chakra (Purity or throat centre)
6. Ajna Chakra (Will or Third Eye centre)
7. Sahasrara Chakra (thousands of petals lotus or crown centre)

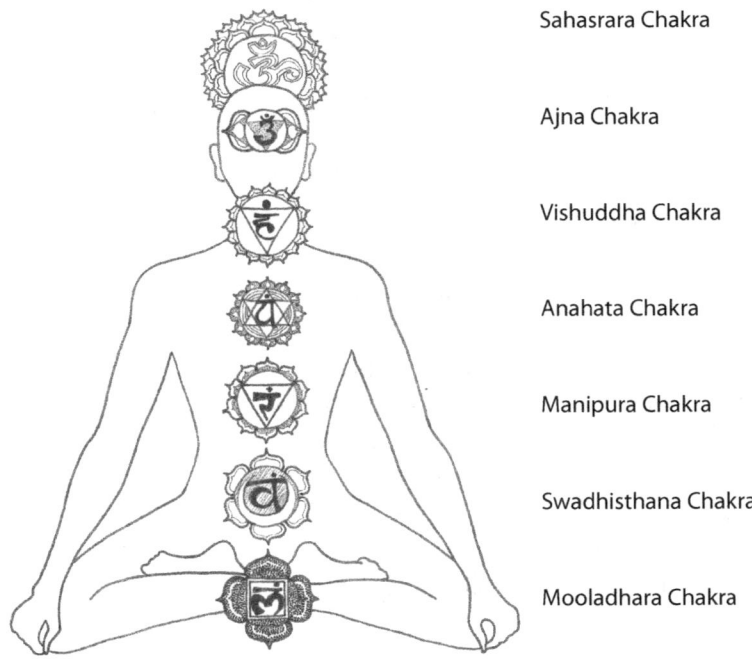

Seven Chakras / Wheels

Do the Chakras exist in Physical Body?

No. Chakras exist in our Pranamaya Kosha or energy body. Chakras are junction or meeting points between our physical body and Pranic Body.

What are the Pancha-Koshas?

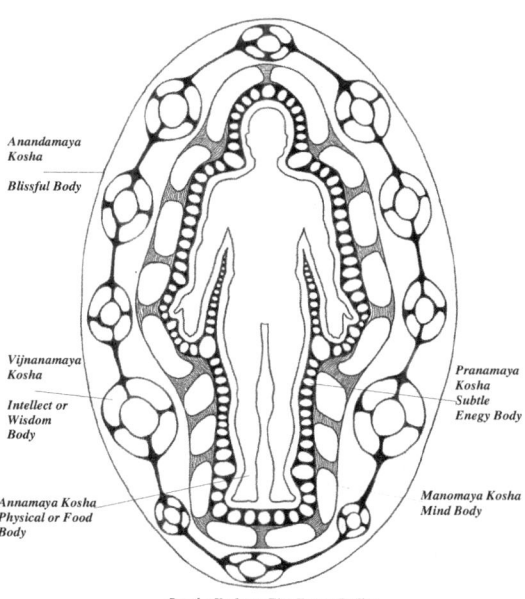

Pancha Kosha or Five Energy Bodies

Yogic science explains our multi-layered existence in the form of Pancha-koshas- five bodies, five layers or sheaths. These are as follows-
1. Annamaya Kosha – food or physical body
2. Pranamaya Kosha – Energy body
3. Manomaya Kosha - Mind-body
4. Vijnanamaya Kosha - Wisdom body
5. Anandamaya Kosha – Bliss body

What is Pranayama Kosha?

Pranamaya Kosha is subtle energy body. This energy is subtlest of energies in the form of electromagnetic force, which vibrates and spins in various wavelengths to support physical and psychological functions. This body has 72,000 Naris. These Naris are the channels for the multiple levels of Prana to flow to different parts of the body.

Energy in Pranamaya Kosha is made of positive and negative ions known as Prana and Apana in Yoga. In this Pranic body, we have our seven chakras. These Chakras are like the little dynamos or transformers. They transform subtle universal pranic force into various sub-pranic energies. These sub-pranic energies from each chakra flow to various parts of the body to sustain all the respective psycho-physiological functions.

What are the Naris?

Naris are energy channels carrying the pranic forces to respective parts of the body like our blood vessels and nerves. Tantra explains 72,000 Naris. Out of these nine are more important regulating some vital functions.

Three Naris is most important for the Yogis. These are Ida, Pingala and Sushumna.

Ida is the left channel. Ida is Silver, feminine, cool, lunar or moon energy. It originates at Mooladhara Chakra and ends in the left nostril.

Pingala is the right channel. Pingala is golden red, masculine, warm, solar energy. Pingala originates at Mooladhara Chakra and ends in the right nostril.

Sushumna is the central channel from Mooladhara flows upward and ends in Anja Chakra. Yogis aim to balance and flow their energies into

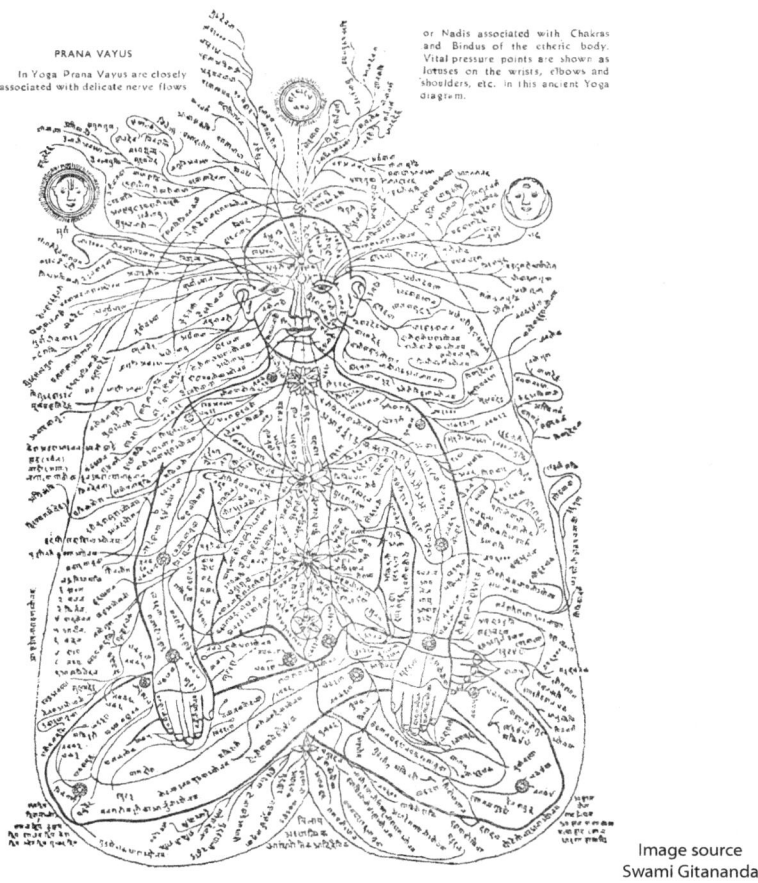

Image source
Swami Gitananda

Sushumna Nari to awaken all the chakras leading the flow into Crown centre.

How are the Chakras associated with Nadis?

Three major Naris along with many minor Naris originate at the Mooladhara Chakra. From here Sushumna Nari flows straight upward, while Ida and Pingala flow upward with crisscrossing each other and Sushumna Nari as the flow upward. You can think of placing number 8 on top of number 8. From Mooladhara to Anja Chakra are the points where these three major Naris are meeting, while Sahashrara or Crown is at the top.

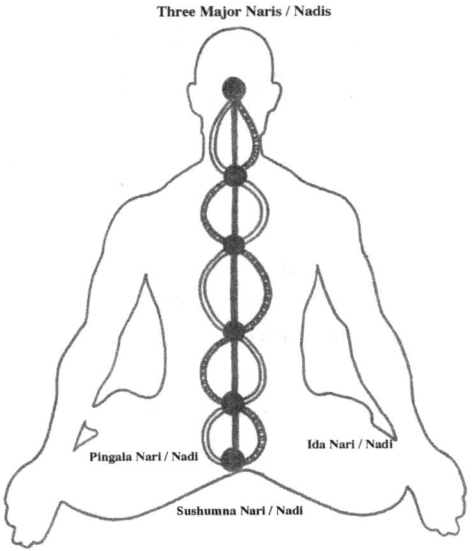

Is there a connection between Chakras and Nerve Plexus?

Yes, each chakra can be associated with a particular nerve plexus. Chakra is a point where all three major Naris are meeting as well as many minor Naris is originating. Similarly, nerve plexus are also points where many nerves are meeting, crisscrossing and arising.

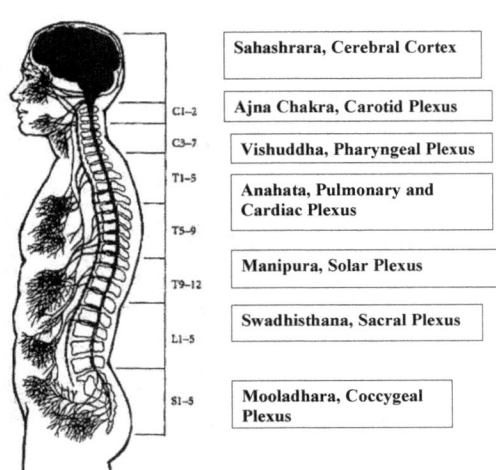

How would we associate Chakras with Endocrine System?

1. Mooladhara Chakra— Adrenal Glands, regulating behaviour patterns life mechanisms.
2. Swadhisthana Chakra — Gonads, or sexual organs.
3. Manipura chakra — Pancreas; governs metabolism.
4. Anahata Chakra — Thymus gland; regulates the immune system.
5. Vishuddha Chakra — Thyroid gland; regulates body temperature and metabolism.
6. Ajna Chakra — Pineal gland; controls biological cycles, including sleep.
7. Sahasrara Chakra — Pituitary gland; produces hormones and governs the function of the other five glands

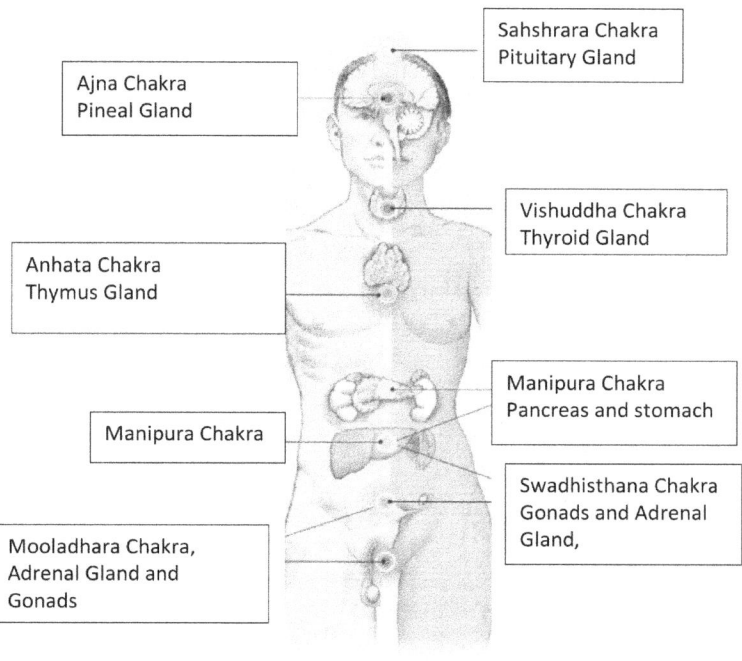

Seven Primary Chakra and their Association with Endocrine Glands

What is Parampara or Lineage?

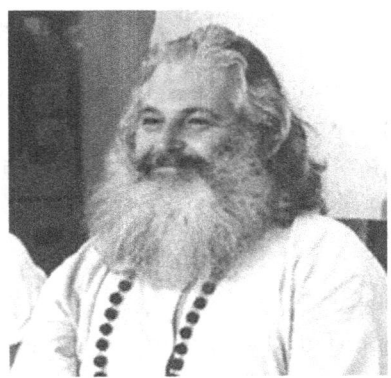

Parampara is a Sanskrit word literally means traditions, practices, or ideas followed in succession from generation to generation. In Yoga, Paramapara refers to the succession of Yoga knowledge from one guru to the next. You can say Parampara is "uninterrupted series," "continuation," or "succession." Guru-Shishya means "from Teacher to Student".

From ancient times Yoga and many other forms of art, dance, skills, and wisdom were passed down by Gurus, self-realised souls or masters to their students. This is really how Vedic, Yogic and Hindu practices, ideas, principals and philosophy evolved and preserved for thousands of years before we have written culture.

Paramapra is a term that is often used in Hinduism as well as in other Indian religions. There are many Paramparais or lineages of Yoga like Natha Parampara, Giri Paramapara, Naga Parampara. They all follow a particular style of yogic practices, kriyas, prakriyas and principals.

What is Bhakti Yoga?

Bhakti Yoga is one of the essential paths of yoga leading to God-Realisation, Self-Realisation or Union with Divine. Hindus believe in many gods or aspects of the divine in human form. But this aspect of offering our life, karma and heart to divine service is practised in every religion. Bhakti Yoga path is to provide all our actions to the supernatural cause, mantra chanting and bhajan singing to evoke and awake divine qualities are the essential practices.

The Nine Limbs of Devotion are as follows-
1. Shravana – "listening" to the ancient scriptures.
2. Kirtana – "singing" devotional songs, usually practised in a call-and-response group format.
3. Smarana – "remembering" the Divine by constantly meditating upon its name and form.
4. Padasevana – "service at the feet" of the Divine, which incorporates the practice of karma yoga (selfless service) with bhakti (devotion).
5. Archana – the "ritual worship" of the Divine through practices such as puja (deity worship), and havan or Homa (fire offering).
6. Vandana – the "prostration" before the image of one's chosen image or representation of the Divine.
7. Dasya – the "unquestioning" devotion of the Divine involving the cultivation of serving the will of God instead of one's ego.
8. Sakhya – the "friendship" and relationship established between the Divine and the devotee.
9. Atmanivedana – the "self-offering" and complete surrender of the self to the Divine.

Swami Sivananda explains benefits of Bhakti Yoga as follows, "Bhakti softens the heart and removes jealousy, hatred, lust, anger, egoism, pride and arrogance. It infuses joy, divine ecstasy, bliss, peace and knowledge. All cares, worries and anxieties, fears, mental torments and tribulations entirely vanish. The devotee is freed from the Samsaric wheel of births and deaths. He attains the immortal abode of everlasting peace, bliss and knowledge".

What is Swara Yoga?

Swara means Sound. Swara Yoga means Union by employing 'sound of breath.' We have three Major Naris or Swaras- Ida, Pingala and Sushumna. Every human being is switching breath and energy flows from one to other Nari or nostril in every 4 to 6 hours. As the Swara or Nari changes, our energy, states of mind and physiology changes too.

A Swara Yogi uses many breathing and pranayama techniques to change flows of energies and prana as the cycles changes to bring balance and harmony. Once all our sub-pranic and pranic forces flow freely in a balanced way, one attains purity and stability of mind and emotions. This path gradually leads to self-realisation or samadhi.

Shiva Swarodaya is vital scripture on Swara Yoga. The breath is essential for human life that ancient Yogis and Rishis found a whole science around breath and Prana in the form of Pranayama Yoga and Swara Yoga. But remember Swara Yoga is not pranayama even though both dealing with Prana.

Swara Yoga emphasises the analysis of the breath and the significance of different Pranic rhythms; whereas, Pranayama involves techniques to redirect, store and enhance Prana. Prana and mind are interlinked with each other as we all know that prana goes where your mind goes. Our mind became restless, agitated and stressed when their lack of prana in quantity or quality. This yoga provides tools to change flows of pranic energy to enhance states of mind and awake true potential energy sleeping in the form of Kundalini.

What are Key Yoga Scriptures?

Many yoga scriptures are detailing various paths or aspects of Yoga. Even though now Yoga Sutras of Patanjali and Hatha Yoga Pradipika are

seen as main or key yoga scriptures, but in reality, if you like to study and practice yoga as complete holistic path then, we need to look into many other scriptures. Here is the list of few-

- ❖ Yoga Sutras of Patanjali
- ❖ Bhagavat Gita- A Dialogue between Lord Krishna and Arjuna
- ❖ Shiva Samhita- a dialogue between Shiva and his wife Shakti on Yoga
- ❖ Hatha Yoga Pradipika- Detailing Hatha Yoga practices to prepare for Raja Yoga.
- ❖ Gheranda Samhita- Also details Hatha Yoga Practices.
- ❖ Yoga Vasishtha- A dialogue between Lord Rama and his Guru Vasishtha.
- ❖ Shiva Swarodaya- the conversation between Lord Shiva and his wife Shakti on the yoga of breath and naris.
- ❖ Yoga Upanishada
- ❖ Vijnana Bhairava Tantra
- ❖ Yoga Chudamani

Yoga Sutras

Yoga is mentioned in many Hindu, Vedic scriptures like Vedas, Upanishads, Bhagavad Gita, etc. But Yoga Sutras of Patanjali is entirely dedicated work on yoga philosophy, each of its limbs, practices, obstacles, etc. Yoga Sutras are a guide map for every human being to reach higher states of mind.

Patanjali compiled and connected many concepts, ideas, practices and principals of yoga as the guide map for Self or Purusha (individual soul) to free itself from worldly mental bondage at attaining Self-realisation or Union with Parmatman (higher self or divine self)

The Sutra means a thread or verse. Yoga Sutras are verses or threads of wisdom. These Yoga Sutras were written in a complex coded Sanskrita

language and to explore and understand them one need to experience each one of them through Sadhana. There is four chapter in yoga sutras containing 195 or 196 Sutras. As in some schools, one of the sutras is divided into two verses. The sutras are divided into four chapters, or padas: samadhi, sadhana, vibhuti, and kaivalya.

Samadhi Pada- The first chapter containing 51 verses is about Samadhi or enlightenment, focusing on states of mind, types of Samadhi, obstacles and tools like abhyasa (practice), and vairagya (detachment).

Sadhana Pada- The second chapter details the Sadhana or practice in forms of eight limbs, karma yoga, kriya yoga and Ashtanga yoga. It describes first six limbs from Yama to Dharana in detail.

Vibhuti Pada- The third chapter is about the siddhis, fruits, power, and manifestation once mastery in practices is achieved. In 56 verses in this chapter, Patanjali explains last two limbs- Dhyana and Samadhi and all the siddhis one attains as milestones on this yogic path. Patanjali advises that Siddhis are just the fruits on the road and not the goal itself.

Kaivalya Pada- The last chapter is about enlightenment, liberation, or moksha. The 34 sutras details about freedom and all the higher states of mind.

Who was Patanjali?

Patanjali considered being lived between 200BC to 2000BC. Patanjali was a great Yogi, attained liberation through following the disciplined path of Yoga.

Gonika, a great Yogini and worshipper of Lord Shiva, was praying for a child to pass on her yogic wisdom. Once she was praying while bathing in the river, she was holding water in her palms (Anjali). A little snake fell her hands as she was praying to Shiva, he blessed that snake to

transformed into a child or yogi, who represents the half snake, half man. Pata means fallen, and Anjali means palms joined together. That's why he was named Patanjali.

Patanjali was represented by a snake because it is the symbol for un-manifested potential energy stored in all of us in the form of Kundalini.

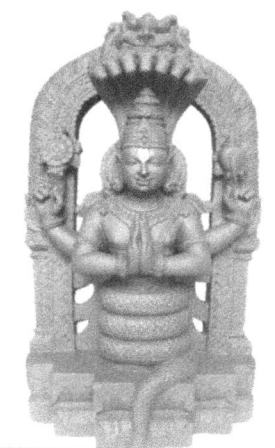

Maharishi Patanjai, Codifier of Yoga Sutras

Bhagavata Gita

The Bhagavad Gita, often known as Gita is one of the key Hindu and Yoga scriptures in poetic forms also known as "Song of the Lord," is part of the Mahabharata, which is an ancient Indian epic.

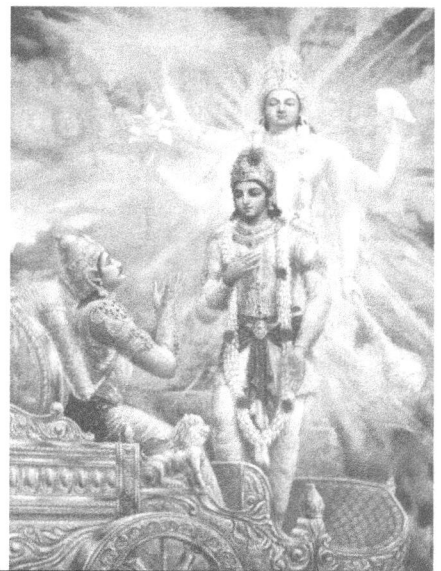

Lord Krishna in discourse with Arjuna on Many Paths of Yoga at the beginning of longest epic war in Indian History

At the beginning of the epic war between Pandavas and Kauravas, Arjuna the greatest warrior and head of Padava army, Arjuna refuses to fight against his relatives and family members. This moment Krishna counsels and teaches Arjuna what is right for him to do as his dharma or duty.

In 18 chapters of Gita, there are 700 verses written in poetic form. These are dialogues between Arjuna and Krishna. Krishna represents the Divine or Supreme Soul (Paramatma),

and Arjuna represents the individual soul (Purusha), and the battle represents the ethical and moral struggles of human mind and life.

Arjuna is filled with doubt and despondency on the battlefield and refuses to fight at the beginning after realising that he is competing against his own family, friends and relatives. He puts his weapons down and askes Krishna, for his advice. Responding to Arjuna's confusion and moral dilemma, Krishna explains to Arjuna his dharma or duties as a warrior and prince, and through the counselling verses of the Gita, awakens wisdom of Arjuna through paths of yoga, jnana, bhakti, Dhyana, and karma yoga.

The Gita details all the psychological tools for the body and mind, including all four paths of yoga, with karma yoga as most important of all in the form of selfless service or performing all the actions devoted to the divine cause.

The Gita is often thought of as a summary of the Upanishads (the Vedanta or essence of the Vedas) and is called "the Upanishad of the Upanishads."

Yoga Vashistha

Yoga Vasishtha is counselling dialogue between Lord Rama in his youth and his Guru Vasishtha. Valmiki between 6th and 14th century wrote it. It contains 19,000 verses. This is written in the form of inspiring stories and fables of great Sages, Rishis and Yogis who attained Liberation through various paths of Yoga.

This work is named after sage Vasishtha, known as the first sage of the Vedanta School by Adi Sankara. It contains six parts. Frist part details Prince Rama's mental and emotional dilemma of confusion, frustration with nature of human life, desires and sufferings. In second chapter it describes quality and character to desire for liberation in the form of Rama.

The third and fourth chapters explain that liberation can be attained through spiritual life, self-effort and understanding universal principals of existence and Truth or Reality. The fifth part describes meditation and its powers of bringing liberation for individual self. In the last chapter, Vasishtha describes states of consciousness and enlightenment to Rama.

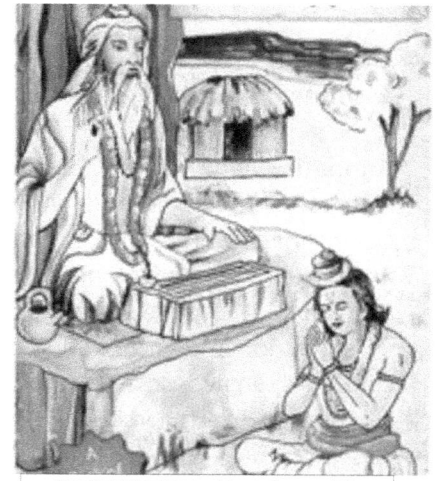

Sage Vashistha giving teachings to Rama on Self-realisation, which are later on compiled as "Yoga Vashistha"

Shiva Samhita

Shiva Samhita is oldest Hatha Yoga Scripture. This scripture is teaching or Lord Shiva to his wife, Paravati or Shakti. This is a complete text on hatha yoga mentioning 84 classical postures, even though it details on four asanas in detail. It describes five types of Prana, Tantra, Mudras and Meditation techniques and yoga philosophy. There was no actual evidence of dates when this scripture was written. Shiva Samhita covers following subjects in detail-

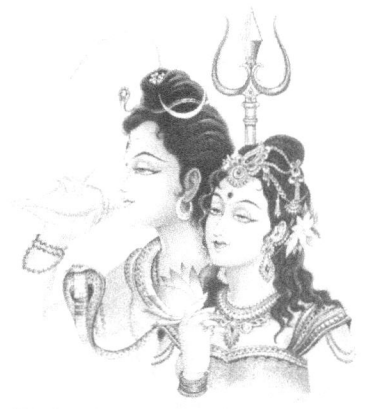

Lord Shiva Who Taught Yoga to His Wife Parvati or Shakti First When She enquired about how to attain Freedom and Samadhi

- Naris, Sushumna, Ida, Pingala
- Prana, ten types of prana
- How to attain success in yoga
- Who is Adhikari or worthy of doing yoga
- The qualities and characters of someone who is worthy of doing yoga

- The signs of someone whose naris (energy channels in the astral body) have been purified by Nari Shodhana (alternate nostril pranayama)
- The obstacles in yoga
- How to attain mastery in yoga
- Mentions 84 asanas (postures) of which only four are described as most important
- describes only Nari Shodhana as pranayama and the method of doing it
- Mantra yoga and Trataka like shadow gazing, sounds

Yoga Chudamani

The Yoga Chudamani Upanishad commentary on the Sama Veda. It means "Crown Jewel of Yoga". It has 121 verses. As it says in the name, it is for Yoga Sadhakas seeking liberation and Samadhi through yoga practice and purification of mind. Yoga Chudamani explains that Yogi should use every breath as Pranayama with mind focussed on Hamsa Mantra. Unconsciously we are chanting this mantra with every breath, meaning "I am Super-Consciousness". This chanting is known as Ajapa Jap. If we focus on this breathing and mantra, it will awake our Kundalini.

This Upanishad explains Naris, specially Sushumna, the central channel and its connection with all the Chakras. Through this Nari, Kundalini energy can flow upward into Sahasrara or crown centre bringing peace, bliss and enlightenment. It opens the doors to realise Higher Self or Param-Brahma. Brahma is universal self, and Para Shakti manifests in the form of Individual Self. All the five elements also manifest from Para-Shakti or creative-mother-energy. This Upanishada also details five elements or tattvas, the four states of consciousness and our body organs and their ruling divine forces. This details part of Pranayama as Pooraka-inhalation, Rechaka- exhalation and Kumbhaka- retention. This Upanishad explains benefits of pranayama, pratyahara and asana too.

Vijnana Bhairava Tantra

Vijana Bhairava Tantra is classical Tantra Yoga text and excellent and typical example of Guru-Shishya system. Here, Guru is the teacher is Lord Shiva, and Shakti or Parwati is Shishya or student. According to many scholars, its written dates can be around 7th century CE. Vijnana means knowledge which comes directly from experience and Bhairava means Supreme Reality or Divine. It is in the form of the dialogue between Shiva and Parwati. She explains her doubts and desires to know how to attain union of Individual Self with Higher Self. The term Shiva is used for Higher and Shakti for Individual Self.

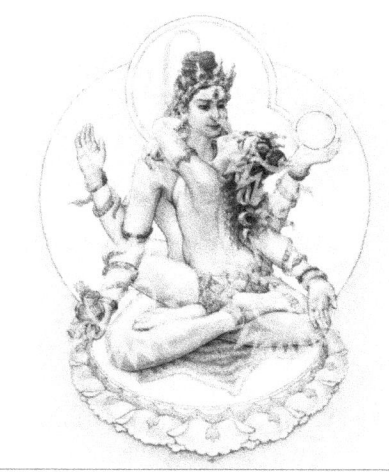

Union of Shiva-Shakti, Prana-Apana, Loma-Viloma, Solur-Lunar, Male-Female energies in form of Shiva-Shakti

Lord Shiva explains how we are under the influence of Maya and duality due to ego and mental bondage. He tells that human mind can not describe Supreme-Consciousness or Reality, but it can be only experienced. This yoga can be practised by using body, mind, breath and subtle life forces- prana. This is the process of self- enquiry to realise Self and Higher Self.

This scripture details 112 techniques of enquiry and meditation to attain Self-realisation. These are aimed to still and focus the mind, awaken kundalini and bring the union of Shiva and Shakti. The techniques include breath awareness, mantra, contemplations and mental energy visualisations. This path has two branches known as North and South. It has more liberal approach compare to other ways of yoga regarding food, lifestyle, sex and material possessions.

Shiva Swarodaya

This scripture is for advance yoga seekers. It is a dialogue between Lord Shiva and his wife, Parvati. This knowledge is being passed down since in Guru-Shishya tradition. This scripture details on Swaras or nostrils, breath and their associations with five elements, states of mind and how to transform our body, mind and life through manipulating and changing our Swaras or nostrils and Breath. It associates right nostril with Pingala and left with the Ida Nari while Sushumna with both nostrils together when the flowing freely.

Hatha Yoga Pradipika

Hatha Yoga Pradipika is one of the most detailed works on Hatha Yoga by Svatmarama Suri. Hatha means forceful, vigorous, zeal, endeavour, steadfast approach to attain the goal of Yoga as Meditation and Samadhi. This literature provides a scientific and experienced approach to asana, pranayama, mudra, bandhas and Dharana practices by many Yogis and master in Hatha Yoga lineage or system.

When the Goddess Parvati, the wife of Lord Siva, enquired to Lord Shiva on how to attain Jnana or Knowledge and experience it for her self to free from suffering and mental whirlpools. She asked how human beings can be free of their physical, psychological and emotional distress. Then Lord Shiva taught her Hatha Yoga science for the holistic development of self.

Parvati passed this knowledge to Brahma, who gave this knowledge to many sages like Narada, Sanka, and Sanatkumara. This Vidya (knowledge) was later in 12th to -15th century was written down as Hatha Yoga Pradipika. Actual reference of teachings goes way far back as even Svatmarama mentions a list of Gurus in his lineage a the knowledge was passed down to him.

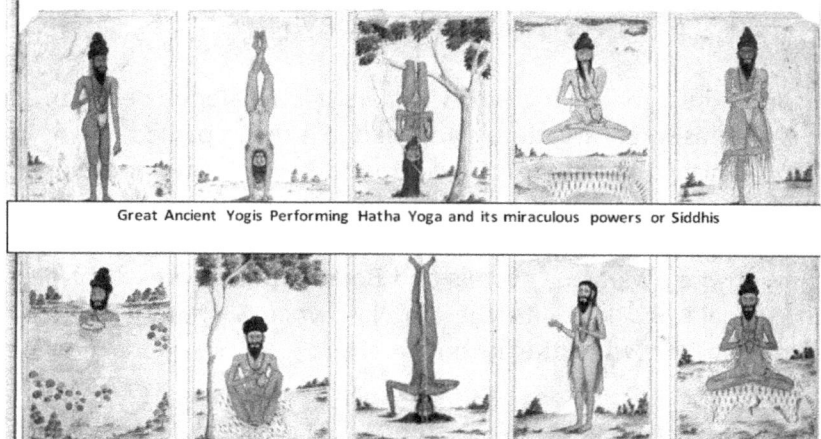

Great Ancient Yogis Performing Hatha Yoga and its miraculous powers or Siddhis

Hatha Yoga is Union a Path of Yoga using Purification Practices, Asana, Mudra, Pranayama, and Dharnas to attain Raja Yoga

From the verses 4-9, Svatmarama invokes and credits this lineage and mentions names of many sages or Yogis through which science hatha yoga was passed down to him.

Hatha Yoga Pradipika is incorporated teachings and practices of Yoga Sutras, Bhagavad Gita and other vital scriptures in its ways. It has all the methods to attain Purity, strengthen, empower and balance of body-mind-energy system to prepare for Raja or Ashtanga Yoga as mentions Svatmarama Suri.

This literature begins with showing gratitude to Lord Shiva who taught this science of Hatha Yoga as the first step of Raja Yoga to his wife, Parwati. Then he closes his work with last verse mentioning that hatha yoga practices serve only to help to prepare for Raja Yoga.

The Pradipika is divided into four parts. The first chapter details Yamas (restraints on behaviour), Niyamas (observances), Asanas (posture) and diet.

The second chapter explains pranayama (enhancement of subtle energy), and the Shat-karmas (internal purification practices).
The third chapter details the mudras (seals, energy gestures), bandhas (locks), the naris (channels of energy through which prana flows) and the kundalini power.

The fourth chapter details about pratyahara (sensory withdrawal), Dharana (concentration), dhyana (meditation), and samadhi (Union).

Gheranda Samhita

"Gheranda Samhita," or "Gheranda's Collection," is one of three important texts on classic Hatha yoga, along with the "Hatha Yoga Pradipika" and the "Shiva Samhita." It was written in Sanskrit in the late 17th century and is sometimes considered to be the most comprehensive of the three texts as it provides a detailed manual for yoga.

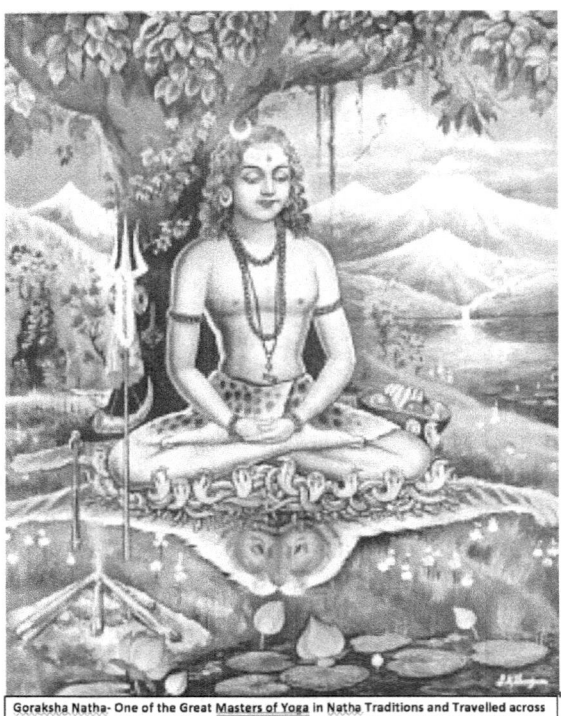

Goraksha Natha- One of the Great Masters of Yoga in Natha Traditions and Travelled across India teaching Hatha Yoga in 11th -12th Century

The yoga text has seven chapters dealing with various limbs of yoga. These seven chapters of "Gheranda Samhita" follow the sevenfold path of yoga, which was taught by the sage Rishi Gheranda to his student, Chanda Kapali.

These seven are:
1. Shatkarmas- Purification of body and mind through six cleansing practices.
2. Asana- for strength, stability and ease of body and channelling the subtle energy- includes 32 postures
3. Mudra- Channeling the energy in various Naris and Chakras to focus the mind and awake consciousness- describes 25 mudras.
4. Pratyahara or sensory withdrawal to concentrate the mind.
5. Pranayama to attain lightness, cleanse naris and enhance Prana. This represents ten classical Pranayama techniques.
6. Dhyana to achieve the realisation of single-pointed awareness.
7. Samadhi or Union – Describes methods of levels of Samadhi.

There is mention of 84 classical Asanas, and out of them, only 32 are described in detail in Gheranda Samhita. Out of these most are seating posture and there is only one standing posture, which is Vrikshasana or Tree Pose.

Yajnavalkya Samhita

Another classical text on Hatha Yoga. The Yogayajnavalikya Samhita is a dialogue between the great sage Yajnavalkya and his learned wife, Gargi. Considered as one of the most learned women of all times, Gargi asks him about how to reach the highest state of consciousness or Samadhi. Yajnavalkya teaches a systematic path of Hatha Yoga to her in twelve chapters in this text.

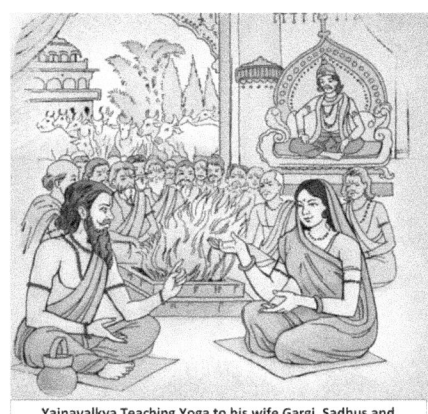

Yajnavalkya Teaching Yoga to his wife Gargi, Sadhus and followers

This Hatha Yoga text named Yoga Yajnavalkya and Yajnavalkya Yoga is also known as Yajnavalkya Gita, Yajnavalkya Samhita and other twelve names. Yajnavalkya is the name of a legendary sage from Vedic times. The Sanskrit word Gita means song, and also translates as words and poem. Samhita means collection.

What are the original dates of Yoga Scriptures?

First to remember that dates of most scripture according to new historians is for the written texts. Yoga and Vedic teachings originally were passed down by the Guru or Teacher directly to Shishya or Student.

Second, our western history believes in humankind to be 7000- to 8000 years old. So for our historians based on modern dating system seems to find it hard to accept anything beyond that timescale.

Third Hindu, Yoga and Samkhya concept of time is not linear as the current time scale; it is spiral. So everything is changing with three motions- Forward, Upward and Inward. To understand dating of yoga scriptures we need to understand Yugas of time cycles in Hindu or Samkhya concepts.

What is the the Four Yugas ?

Each yuga is an age with specific characteristics in which incarnations of Vishnu the sustainer or preserver happens. The four Yugas make up a cycle called Divya-Yuga, which lasts 4,320,000 years. One thousand of these Yugas equal to one day of Brahma, which is known as a Kalpa. Brahma's lifespan is 100 years of his time. In each Yuga, there is a specific process of self-realisation (Yuga Dharma).

SATYA YUGA - (krta-yuga): the golden age or time of Truthfulness lasts 1,728,000 years. The process of self-realisation in this Yuga is the meditation on the divine. During this Yuga, the majority of people live

in harmony, love, peace and truthfulness. Average lifespan is 100,000 years. Goodness and darkness is 80-20 ration.

TRETA YUGA - also known as the silver age, is 1,296,000 years long and the process of self-realisation is the performance of yajnas(sacrificial service). The average lifespan is 10,000 years, and the divine and dark qualities are in 60-40 ratio. The Varna-Ashrama-dharma is introduced in this phase.

DVAPARA YUGA - or the bronze age, lasts 864,000 years and the process of self-realisation is the worship (Bhakti) and Karma (selfless action). Here the Goodness and darkness are in 50-50 ration, and lifespan is 1000 years.

KALI YUGA - the iron age of hypocrisy and darkness lasts 432,000 years. Lord Krishna appeared in His original, transcendental form right before the beginning of Kali Yuga. The process of self-realisation is Satsanga, Hatha and Raja Yoga. Lifespan is reduced to 100 years, and by the end of Kali Yuga, it will cut down to 20 years. Here the ratio of divine and darkness is 20-80.

Indian Mythological History and Scriptures

Indian or Santana Dharma has a vibrant culture and history dating back from Satyuga all the way to Kaliyuga, Rama was one of the Vishnu incarnations happened in Satyuga. Krishna, another incarnation of Vishnu, happened in Dvapara Yuga. Original dates of Ramayana can be dated between 1,728,000 and 1,296,000 years old. These scriptures are Ramayana, and Yoga Vasishtha.

Then we have Lord Krishna in Dwapara Yuga and Mahabharata, and Bhagavat Gita should be dated in this time phase. This is just an example how old original teachings are.

The dates of this scripture we read now are only for the time when they were written in the present form. But originally lessons were being passed down in oral traditions, and hence modern historical dating of these scriptures is not fair or accurate.

Did only men practice yoga as we hear from many modern yoga teachers?

No. Yoga was practised by men and women equally. There has never been gender difference on the evolutionary path of liberation. If you study most Hatha Yoga Scriptures, there is enough evidence of yoga being taught to women.

Hatha Yoga Pradipika, Gheranda Samhita and Shiva Samhita mention that Parwati, wife of Shiva askes him to show her path of yoga. All three scriptures are dialogues between two of them, which clearly states that women were practising yoga too. Similarly, Yajnavalkya Samhita was first taught by Yajnavalkya to his wife, Gargi.

There are many stories of enlightened women yoginis in various scriptures like Leela in Yoga Vasishtha, Gargi in Yajnavalkya, Parwati or Shakti in Hatha Yoga Pradipika, Shiva Samhita, Vijnana Bhairava Tantra, etc.

The Hatha Yoga Pradipika, Gheranda Samhita, Shiva Samhita, and Yajnavalkya Samhita mention benefits of asana, pranayama and mudras to reduce the pain of menstrual cycle, improve fertility or health of uterus in women. This evidence shows us that yoga was practised by women too.

Natha Guru Gorksha Nathji states that "oh dear men and women if you want to remain healthy, learn to breathe deep and practice Pranayama."

Did ascetics or spiritual seekers only practice yoga?

No. Even though it seems primary goal of yoga is self-realisation, but yoga is also a path to live, grow and evolve for household people. Yamas and Niyamas, Asana and Pranayama, were practised widely across India by men and women. Again many scriptures detail therapeutic benefits of Asana, Shata Karmas, Pranayama, Mudra and moral and ethical principals of yoga, which indicates clearly that households also practised yoga.

What is an Ashram?

The ashram is an institute or home of a Guru or teacher where his or her followers or students can come and live to learn and practice yoga. It was a safe space created to accommodate teachings in Ancient India. Nowadays we relate ashram to a religious yoga, spiritual place or a cult. Initially, Ashrams in India was a Sanskrit term being used for the educational place like modern schools or university.

We have little ashrams or Yoga Shalas across India from north to south. These places are open for Sadhus, Monks, Yogis or teachers to go and live anytime they need to. Here local villagers and residents will fulfil day to day needs, and in exchange, these masters will pass their yoga vidya to them. Satsang, Kirtans, Hatha Yoga Shala, are some typical examples of ashram events. I have lived as a Natha Sadhu for two plus years and enjoyed my sadhana and teaching.

Is it true that first Hatha Yoga was taught in 1918 in India?

No. I have heard about this quite a few times recently. Maybe it was the first time when some taught a hatha yoga session with the registration form, health and safety, etc. or prepaid fees. As I mentioned above Hatha Yoga was taught in ashrams or Hatha Yoga Shalas across India.

Some ashrams I have been known to be 1000s of years old. Just remember all these ashrams were being held or run by general household Indians. You might argue that it was the first time someone taught out of ashram, but these Sadhus, Yogis and yoga masters travelled across the country many times and spread their teachings and knowledge where ever they stayed. It can also be seen as finding a date when someone first time has education out of a school or university as they are there for providing education.

What are Eight Limbs of Yoga in Summary?

Ashtanga or Raja Yoga in Yoga Sutras, Samkhya Yoga and other scriptures describe eight limbs or steps of yogic evolution. It is a guide map for everyone seeking for self-realisation. These eight limbs are as follows-

Yamas- Yamas or restrains on our animal nature is the first limb. These are Ahimsa (non-violence), Satya (truth), Asteya (non-stealing), Brahmacharya (energy discipline), and Aparigraha (detachment). These Yamas teach us how to fulfil our basic needs without causing pain to others.

Niyamas- Niyama or observances are the second limbs of Ashtanga Yoga. These are Saucha (purity), Samtosha (contentment), Tapah (austerity), Swadhyaya (self-study) and Iswara Pranidhana (offering service to divine cause). These Niyamas are to help us become a good human being and evolve.

Asana- Asana, Posture, Pose, or a firm seat is the third limb of Raja Yoga. This limb is to attain health, strength and ease of body and mind to sit comfortably for Pranayama and further limbs.

Pranayama- Pranayama generally known as breathing exercises is forth limb of Raja Yoga. This limb is to purify our subtle energy, mind and naris to attain enhanced pranic energy.

Pratyahara- Pratyahara is a door to higher yoga, concentration, meditation and self-realisation. This is to withdraw or senses and focus them on external or distracted focus to internal or single-pointedness. Pratyahara is generally translated as withdrawal of senses.

Dharna- Dharna is the sixth limb, and it means concentration. Dharna is to focus our mind on one point. There are many dharna or concentration practices described in various scriptures.

Dhyana- Dhyana or meditation is the seventh limb of Raja Yoga. This is not something we can practice, but it is a state of single-pointed mind, where mind merges entirely into the point of concentration or dharna.

Samadhi- Last and eight limbs of Ashtanga Yoga, every Yogi seeks to attain means Union, Liberation, Enlightenment or self-realisation.

What is Yama?

Yama is a Sanskrita term, means restraint or to bring under control our animal behaviour pattern. We all have three basic biological needs and would do anything to fulfil them unless we are trained otherwise. These biological needs are hunger, thirst and sex. Pancha Yamas are moral or ethical practices on how to achieve these needs without causing harm or taking advantage.

Yamas help us to fulfil all our requirements with following principles -
1. Without causing damage (Ahimsa, Non-violence).
2. Without being dishonest (Satya, truth)
3. Without stealing or taking what does not belong to us (Asteya, non-stealing)
4. Not accumulating or hanging on to things we don't need (aparigraha, non-greed)
5. Control or discipline of our sensual energy (brahmacharya, the discipline of physical energy).

What are Pancha Yamas?

Pancha Yamas are Ahimsa (non-violence, non-harm), Satya (truth, honesty), Asteya (non-stealing), Brahmacharya (the discipline of sensual energy) and Aparigraha (non-accumulation, non-greed).

Ahimsa

Ahimsa is first of the five Yamas which means restraining from causing any harm or pain to anyone through any mean like physical, verbal, mental. Ahimsa is not only not causing damage but also not allowing others to cause harm to you either. Vedas explains Ahimsa as our highest duty or Dharma (Ahimsa parmo dharmah). In Bhagavat Gita Lord Krishna also explains to Arjuna that we must protect others if we can do in any way possible.

Satya

Satya means truth or honesty. Abstaining from any lies, dishonesty and manipulation is Satya. Yogic Truth is not only what we know or have learned, but it is what we have experienced ourselves. As a yoga Sadhaka, what you learn, you should practice and experience it to know the truth. The highest practice of Satya is not manipulating our experiences and understanding of facts we know. The Vedic concept of Satya is "speak the truth, speak the sweet truth, don't speak the bitter truth". Ammaji Meenakshi Devi adds another one to this –"Speak the bitter truth in the sweetest possible way."

Asteya

Asteya is third of Pancha Yamas means non-stealing or not taking anything does not belong to us. Stealing other's thoughts, ideas or concepts are becoming common these days. Even so, many new yoga branches or modernised yoga teachings promoted without referencing to India or Hindu / Sanatan Dharma. Stealing someone's time which can be used for their personal development of evolution.

Brahmacharya

Brahmacharya translated as chastity or restraint of any sexual activity. This can not be, true in its real sense as the Yogic idea is based on four phases of life and one of them is being household which involves having family and kids. Most of ancient Rishis and Gurus were married. So to me, Brahmacharya is control or discipline of our sensual energy and drives and how to fulfil them.

Aparigraha

The fifth and last of Pacha Yama is Aparigraha means non-greed or non-accumulation. Living a simple life with taking "what we need" as well as letting go of "things we don't need" is Aparigraha. Our possessiveness has grown so deep now that we are even holding on to our problems and pain. People say my blood pressure, diabetes, heart problem, etc., etc. is extreme of attachment to anything or everything.

What are the Panch Niyamas?

Niyamas are the second limb of Ashtanga or Raja Yoga. Niyama means rules or ethics we need to follow. These are the further extension of Yamas or ethical values. Yogis find these Yamas and Niyamas as tools to purify our body, mind, emotions, behaviour patterns and channel our drive forces in search of health, happiness and evolution.

Niyamas are five observations a Sadhaka need to adhere to for spiritual growth. Yamas to restrain our animal nature while Niyamas are the practices to become a good human being. These are to maintain the purity of our body, mind, attitude, karma and drive forces. These Niyamas help us keep a clean, healthy and positive environment around us.

Shaucha (purity)

This is first of the Niyamas. Shaucha means purity or cleanliness. Hatha Yoga describes Shata Karmas in detail for purification of our body and mind. The purity or cleanliness of our body, surrounding, house, clothes,

food, mind, thoughts, and environment is vital for human health and happiness.

Samtosha (contentment)
Samtosha is being happy with fruits of our actions as well as not desiring for what we don't have and not holding on to what we do not need. Yogis explain that true happiness is in contentment in life. Lord Krishna tells that we need to do our best and leave the rest. Contentment is also not worrying about fruits and not judging or comparing ourselves with material possessions. Material bondage brings fear; fear causes pain, anger and suffering. Even some time being self-satisfied with our actions once we have done our best, not pushing ourselves beyond our limits in the day to day life.

Tapas (austerity or practice)
Tapas is intense self-discipline and following all the yogic practices with willpower. Tapas is doing what you need to do to grow spiritually. Tapas also means fire or putting our body and mind through that intense heat of yogic sadhana to burn all the mental, emotional and spiritual impurities. Tapas leads us in controlling all our mental and emotional whirlpools and awaken our consciousness and kundalini power. Tapas build the willpower and personal strength to help us become more dedicated to our practice of yoga.

Swadhyaya (self-study)
Swadhyaya is the ability to seek for our true divine nature through introspection. It is looking inward to see how we act, react and respond to all the life events, and practices we do. We get a thought, and in response to that we get another thought, and gradually it becomes a series of thoughts which can be positive or negative. All this goes on our body has to also respond to each one of them. If you think happy thoughts, your body will feel light and full of prana. If you are thinking negative or stressful thoughts, your body also feels tensed and tired.

This Swadhyaya, in the beginning, is to keep witnessing every thought and their reaction and response. Gradually Swadhyaya is cultivating

positive thoughts and ideas, focussing on universal principals of prana, life, soul and divine though contemplations.

Ishvara Pranidhana (faith, devotion)
Ishvara Pranidhana is the last of Pancha NIyamas which is practised through dedication, devotion, and faith in divine and offering all our actions and fruits to the divine cause. It is the change of transformation of our attitude from "what do I want? `What do I get? To What can I do? What can I give?". This is fruitless action or Karma. This is also seeing life and every event as a divine blessing. We all have this life to grow and evolve, and universe or divine has given this beautiful opportunity to work out our karma and fulfil our Dharma or duties.

Do I need to practice Yamas and Niyamas Universally?

Yes. Patanjali mentions that Yamas and Niyamas are to be followed universally in reference to area, cast, colour and species. We need to treat every life with equal respects, love and care.

What are Shata Karmas?

Hatha Yoga science teaches us six cleansing practices to purify our body and mind. These are necessary to get rid of all the toxins and impurities as otherwise, they will keep causing health issues, negative thoughts and emotions. These are as follows-
1. Neti: nasal cleaning, including Jala neti and sutra neti.
2. Dhauti: the cleansing of the digestive tract.
3. Nauli: abdominal massage.
4. Basti: colon cleansing.
5. Kapalbhati: purification and vitalisation of the frontal lobes.
6. Trataka: gazing to purify our focus.

What is Asana?

Asana is the third limb of Raja Yoga, which means a seat, state or being, or throne. Patanjali describes asana as "sthiram sukham asanam" means "steady, stable, pleasant posture is Asana." Asana or posture is for achieving a healthy body and healthy mind so one can be comfortable in one position or asana for meditation and other higher practices. Asana helps us to attain union of body, mind and breath.

Why do we Practice Asana?

Asana has many aspects and benefits for everyone depending on what they are looking for. Most of us might follow or practice asana for strength, flexibility, relaxation, better sleep, heal injuries, health benefits, etc., etc.

Others practice asana for their psychological and mental benefits to attain calmness and serenity of mind. Yogis follow and practice Asana to enhance the quality of prana, purify naris, open chakras and transcend energy flow from lower to higher chakras.

How does Asana helps dealing with stress?

Our body naturally like to come to its state of ease or balance known as homeostasis. Due to the busy life, stress, and burden, our body and mind get confused and start to remain in tension most of the time. The concept of classical asana is based on spanda-nispanda (doing-letting go and being). So you do your ASANA- stretch, twist, or bend as part of the action, then you let go and relax to achieve the state of ease to retrain our body-homeostasis system. This gradually builds us to help our body and mind to relax even in stressful situations.

What is Vinyasa or Kriya in Hatha Yoga?

Hatha Yoga work has always been mix and balance of dynamic and static practices. Hatha Yoga in dynamic form is commonly known as Vinyasa or Kriya. A vinyasa of Kriya is set of Asanas with movement from one pose to other poses with conscious breathing and awareness not only about body and breath but also on every transition and transformation at body, mind and energy levels. It can be as simple as simple as leg or hand lift with breath and awareness, or it can be as complex as extended Rishikesh Suriya Namaskar with 84 classical postures in the flow or movement.

What does Suriya Namaskar mean?

Suriya is Sanskrita term of Sun and Namaskar is for salutation or greeting. Suriya Namaskars are typical examples of Hatha Yoga Vinyasa or Kriyas. In generally used as warm-up or preparatory for asana. In our tradition, we have many variations of sun-salutations with various energy, attitude, chakras, naris, strength and flexibility ideas. Some of them are like Aruna Suriya Namaskar, Vedic Suriya Namaskar, Rishikesh Suriya Namaskar, etc. Some schools follow them with breath, others also follow them with Suriya Mantras or seed mantras for the sun.

How many Classical Asanas are there?

Various scriptures describe the various number of postures like 84, 32 and out of them four meditation postures are most important. These are Sukhasana, Vajrasana, Padmasana and Siddhasana. Hatha-Yoga, Gheranda Samhita and Yajnavalkya are some of the texts have great detail on Asana and Mudras. Asana is to refine, awaken and channel or gross energies to subtle energies.

Yoga in Modern Age

In recent times or last 50-60 years the meaning of yoga and followings of yoga has shifted in many perspectives significantly. The practice of Asana, hatha yoga, pranayama has become the synonym of yoga now. That is what most people think of yoga nowadays, doing one or other forms of physical exercise.

The deep, eternal and true essence of yoga has been misconceived/ misinterpreted and limited to a few exercises undermining its spiritual dimension. The relative position of the postures (asanas), has become the top priority and primary practice. This is misleading many yoga seekers to that the term 'Yoga' refers to physical postures only, as well as, a few breathing exercises on the name of pranayama and that the goal of these is nothing but physical fitness.

What is Pranayama?

Forth, the limb of Ashtanga yoga is pranayama. Prana means the subtlest form energy which exists before creation, it exists right through the existence, and it will exist at the end. We are continuously exchanging between individual prana and universal prana through our breath, drinks, food and sensory inputs. As breathing is one of the most common and continuous exchange, yogis used breath as a tool to purify, control and enhance the prana to awaken our potential energy, sleeping in the form of kundalini otherwise.

What is Prana?

Prana is universal catalytic force or energy in the form of subtlest electromagnetic ions. This is the mother or creative energy from which everything -living and non-living matter manifests. Einstein also explains same as the law of energy conservation. This energy is

transforming dynamically in many forms, but still, it remains conserved. Like in a swing motion energy changing from potential to kinetic and kinetic to potential energy.

This eternal divine force is cleaver, intelligent and holds all the universal laws of creation, sustain, and evolution like the seeds of a flower or a plant. The seed holds all the DNA formulas or intelligence on how to utilise all the elements to grow into what it meant to be.

What are the Pancha Vayus?

Universal Prana, transforms into Sub-Pranic energies known as Vayus for all our psycho-somatic and spiritual functions. These are five, and each one is associated with a particular chakra and flow in the specific direction in various parts of body organs they are associated with.

Here is the table-

Pancha Prana or Prana Vayus

Vayu	Body Region	Movement	Area Between	Function
1. Prana	heart region	Upward	larynx and diaphragm	breathing, food and liquid swallowing
2. Apana	lower regions	Downward	Navel and perineum	Elimination of urine, faeces, gas, wind, sexual fluids, menstrual blood, and the faetus at the time of birth
3. Samana	Digestive area	Lateral moving	Diaphragm and navel	All digestive functions and also the heating and cooling of the body
4. Udana	Peripheral parts	Spiraling	Above the larynx and also the arms	Brain and all sensory receptors- eyes, ears, nose, tongue and skin are governed as well as three organs of action-speech, hands and feet
5. Vyana	All-pervasive	All directions	Whole body	Reserve force for all four and maintenance of their depletion, regulation of physical movements

What are the associations of Pancha Vayus with Chakras?

Below is the table of Prana-Vayus and their association with chakras and Pancha-mahabhutas (five elements).

Prana Vayu	Chakra	Element
Prana Vayu	Ajna Chakra	Vayu, Air
Apana	Mooladhara	Prathvi, Earth
Samana	Manipiur	Agni, Fire
Udana	Vishuddha	Akasha, Ether
Vyana	Swadhisthana	Jala, Water

Is Pranayama Breathing exercise?

No. Even though we use breath or breathing exercises as the primary tool, but Pranayama is the enhancement of quality, quantity and vibration of Prana. We use breath as the tool in various rhythms, nostrils, lengths and sounds to tune into multiple bio-rhythms, energy flows, and chakras to purify our body, mind and naris, which allows the prana to flow freely to bring lightness, health and happiness.

Why do we practice Pranayama?

Pranayama can be taken as practice for its benefits to improve breathing, enhance mental clarity, balance our energy flows, purify the body-mind system, recharge pranic body, activate or recharge chakras and bio-energy flows, etc., etc.

Classically Pranayama as forth limb of Raja Yoga is to purify of body, mind and naris to prepare for higher or internal limbs of yoga like concentration, meditation and samadhi.

Pranayama according to Ammaji Meenakshi Devi Bhavanani

Ancient Sanskrit sources proclaim that Pranayama is a "holy science" leading to inner spiritual development. "Prana is the fundamental basis of whatever is, was, and will be." (Atharvaveda XI, IV, 10: XI, IV, 15) "Pranayama is a technique bringing under control all that is connected with Prana (Vital Force). (Vishnu Puranam, VI, VII, 40) Whatever our source, the ancient Rishis all agree that there is vital energy called "Prana" and that it can be controlled, "Ayama." The science of this control is "Pranayama".

What are four aspects of Pranayama?

Pranayama has four parts where universal and individual prana finds their connection, flow and union between each other. These are as follows-

Sanskrita	English	Type
Puraka	Inhalation	Prana
Anter Kumbhaka	Hold in	Vidharana
Rechaka	Exhalation	Prachardana
Bahira Kumbhaka	Hold out	Apana

For advance Sadhaka there is also firth part known as Sunyaka where breath naturally ceases or prana completely absorbs in its source or point of origin.

What is classical Pranayamas according to Hatha Yoga Pradipika?

Hatha Yoga Pradipika details following eight pranayamas in chapter 2.

Sitkari Pranayama
Verse 54: "Then Sitkari (is described) Make a hissing sound with the mouth (while inhaling air) and exhale only through the nostrils. By the Yoga consisting of repeated practice of this, one becomes the second god of beauty (Kamadeva)"

Verse 55: "He becomes an object of high regard amongst the circles of Yogins; he can create and destroy; neither hunger nor thirst, somnolence or indolence arise (in him)."

Verse 56: "By this practice strength of body is gained, and the Lord of Yogins becomes surely free of afflictions of every kind on this earthly sphere.

Sitali Pranayama
Verse 57: "Then Sitali (is described) (Protruding the tongue a little outside the lips) Inhale with the tongue (curled up to resemble a bird's beak) and perform Kumbhaka as before. Then the intelligent (practitioner) should slowly exhale the air through the nostrils."

Verse 58: This Kumbhaka named Sitali destroys diseases of the abdomen and spleen and also fever, biliousness, hunger, thirst, and (the bad effects of) poisons."

Bhramari Pranayama
Verse 68: "Here Bhramari is described. Breathing in rapidly with a resonance resembling the sound of a bee, exhale slowly, making the humming sound of a female bee. By the Yoga, which consists in practising thus, there arises an indescribable bliss in the hearts of the best amongst the Yogins.

Bhastrika Pranayama
Verse 59: "Then Bhastrika: When the two feet are placed upon (opposite) thighs, that is the Padmasana which destroys all ill effects."

Verse 60-61: Having assumed Padmasana properly, with the neck and abdomen in line, the intelligent (practitioner) should close the mouth and breathe out the air through the nostrils with effort, till it is felt to resound in the heart, throat and up to the skull. Then air should be inhaled rapidly till it touches the lotus of the heart.

Verse 62-63: Again he should exhale in the same manner and inhale thus again and again. Even as the blacksmith works his bellows with speed, he should with his mind, keep the Prana in his body (consistently) by moving. When tiredness is felt in the body, he should breathe in through right nostril.

Verse 64: After the interior of the body is quickly filled with air, the nose should be closed tightly with the thumb, the ring finger, and the little finger.

Verse 65: Having performed as prescribed, the breath should be exhaled through the left nostril. This removes (disorders rising from) excess of wind, bile and phlegm and increases the (digestive) fire in the body.

Murcha Pranayama
Verse 69: Then Murccha is described. At the end of inhalation, very firmly assuming Jalandhara Bandha, exhale breath slowly. This is called "Murccha" as it reduces the mind to a state of inactivity and confers happiness.

Chapter Five V.7: Having performed Kumbhaka with comfort, let him withdraw the mind from all objects and fix it in the space between the eyebrows. This causes fainting of mind and gives happiness. For, by this joining the Manas with the Atma, the bliss of Yoga is certainly obtained.

Suriya Bhedana

Verse 48. Then Surya Bhedana is described. Assuming an Asana on a comfortable seat, the Yogi should slowly draw the air outside through the right Nadi (Pingala)

Verse 49: Then he should practise Kumbhaka, restraining the breath to the utmost till it is felt from the hair (on the head) to the ends of the nails (in the toes, that is, pervading the whole body). Then, he should slowly exhale through the left Nadi (Ida)

Verse 50: This excellent Surya Bhedana should, again and again, be practised as it purifies the brain, destroys diseases rising from the excess of wind, and cures maladies caused by worms (bacteria).
(Before this Swatmarama Suri generally says about Pranayama Verse.

45: At the end of inhalation, (Puraka) the Jalandhara Bandha should be practised. At the end of Kumbhaka, and at the beginning of exhalation (Rechaka), Uddiyana Bandha should be practised.)

Verse 46: Contracting the throat (in the Jalandhara Bandha) and the anus (in Mula Bandha) at the same time, and by drawing back the abdomen (in Uddyana Bandha) the Prana flows through Sushumna Nadi (Brahma Nadi)

Ujjayi Pranayama

Verse 51: Now Ujjayi is described. Closing the mouth, draw in air slowly through both nostrils till the breath is felt to be sonorous from the throat to the heart.
Verse 52: Perform Kumbhaka as before and exhale through Ida. This removes disorders in the throat caused by phlegm and stimulates digestive fire.

Verse 53: It puts an end to the diseases of the Nadis and the Dhatus as also dropsy. Walking or standing this Ujjayi should be practised.

Plavini Pranayama
Verse 70: Then Plavini is described. Owing to the air, which has been abundantly drawn in, completely filling the interior, the Yogi floats easily, even in deep waters, like a lotus leaf.

Dr Swami Gitananda Giri Ji on Pranayama
"God is breath" is the oldest Sanskrit writing. Etymologists have stated that our Sanskrit word "Brahman" is a synonym for "breath." "Breath is life; life is breath." The Hebrew mystic states, "God breathed into Man the Breath of Life, and he became a living Breath (Soul)." To be "in breath" is to be "in God." The Greek word for the taking-up of the breath, "in spiro" means to be "in Spirit." "Ex-spiro", the expelled breath, is "to be parted from God." The taking of breath is a holy, divine function and those who aspire to Divinity must master the Kriyas and Prakriyas of Pranayama, the Yoga of Controlled Breathing.

How in depth is Hatha Yoga Science in Gitananda Tradition according to Ammaji Meenakshi Devi?

The Eight Classical Pranayamas detailed in Hatha Yoga Pradipika are considered by the Rishi Culture Ashtanga Yoga Tradition of Dr Swami Gitananda to be relatively advanced practices, which should be taught only after basic training in proper breathing is given, especially through the Hathenas, or Forcing Techniques which condition the body to deep, controlled, conscious breathing. Yogamaharishi Dr Swami Gitananda Giri was the lineage holder of the Yoga Bengali Tantric tradition of Yogamaharishi Kanakananda Bhrigu. This tradition is part of the Dakshina Marga Tantra, which aims at the control of Shakti through an elaborately structured lifestyle, and cultivation of hundreds of Yoga techniques. In this tradition more than 375 Asanas, Kriyas, Mudras, Bandhas and cleansing practices are taught along with more than 120 Pranayamas, designed to cleanse, purify, strengthen and sensitise the body, emotions and mind, making the human being a fit vehicle of the Divine Spirit.

As Swamiji often said, "God breathed the Breath of Life into the man, and he became a living soul. Now, it is our duty as evolving beings to guard and cherish that Breath of Life as our spiritual treasure. We must deepen it, lengthen it, control it, expand it and become conscious of it and its potentiality to link us with our Highest Nature. That is the real Pranayama, the ancient spiritual Science of Vital Control."

Is there the connection between mind and prana?

Yes. In Geeta, Lord Krishna states that the mind is the vehicle of prana. Thus your awareness goes where your thought goes. Your mind goes where your awareness goes, and there goes the prana. Therefore the mind or the thoughts and emotions need the prana or the conscious to travel in and out. Those who do mental work at the end of the day, they feel more tired in comparison to those who are doing the only physical job. Why? This happens because our psychological and emotional processes consume more prana than the physical process. So be careful and aware of what you think and what you feel. You need to be mindful of the mental and emotional process to check and remove them.

What is the success in Pranayama?

Success in pranayama is entirely dependent upon direct experiential sensitivity to and conscious relationship with the prana and its source. After practice, one realises that the wavelike operations of the mind (cit-vrtti) are dependent upon the actions of the prana. The vibrations of the prana are available through the vibrations in the air. By refining the air and prana and by making them highly subtle, eventually, the mind opens up to its vast potential. This requires a requisite amount of direct experiential sensitivity of inner wisdom. As the mind empties, as the breath empties, as the prana becomes most subtle (empty), as the mental objects dissolve, then the total purity of mind is attained and samadhi dawns as we are filled with Divine vibration (spanda).

What is Pratyahara?

The term pratyahara is derived from two Sanskrit terms, Prati and Ahara. Ahara means "food," or "anything we take into ourselves from the outside." Prati is a preposition meaning "against" or "away." Pratyahara means literally "control of Ahara," or "gaining mastery over external influences from stimulants." Ahara is termed for all the external stimulants and distractions which attracts our sense organs outward, and gradually our mind flows out and results in whirlpools or Chitta-vrittis.

Pratyahara is like a turtle withdrawing its limbs into its shell in case of danger or attacks and keeps itself safe as the shell is strong to protect its soft limbs and body. The turtle's shell is the manas or consciousness, and the senses are the limbs. The term is usually translated as "withdrawal from the senses," but it is the withdrawal of senses from the external stimulants, which results in an introvert flow of prana or vital energy and finally rests in its Chitta or consciousness which is state of "sensory withdrawal".

Is Pratyahara Bahiranga or Antaranga Yoga?

As the fifth of the eight limbs, pratyahara stands in central place. Some yogis describe it among the outer aspects of yoga / Bahiranga yoga, while others with the inner aspects of yoga / Antaranga yoga. Pratyahara is the key between the outer and inner aspects of yoga; it is entry and exit; external to internal and vice versa aspects of yoga. It teaches us how to move in and out from one to the other.

What are senses?

The mind is in constant motion and is affected in every moment by all the mental, emotional activities, images, sounds and other sensual perceptions, which it perceives through the senses. This is inherent nature of mind

Yoga philosophy describes 11 Indriyas or sense organs. The 11 Indriyas are further divided into five Jnanendriyas, five Karmendriyas, and manas (mind). While Samkhya Yoga describes 14 indriyas- five Jnanendriyas, five Karmaendriyas, buddhi, ahamkara, Prakriti and Purusha.

What are five Jnanendriyas?

Jnanendriya originated from the roots jnana (wisdom), and Indra who is the God of the 'sensory', or heaven in Hinduism. These are the 5 (Pancha) physical sense organs — these enable one to perceive the world around them. These are:
- Shotra — ears
- Chakshu — eyes
- Grahna — nose
- Jivha — tongue
- Tvak — skin

What are five Karmendriyas?

Karmendriya means 'organ of action' – that which facilitates our sensory contact with the outer world — or that which enables us to interact with the material objects of the world. These five organs of action are:
- Pada (feet) — for locomotion
- Pani/hasta (hands) — for dexterity
- Payu (rectum) — for excretion
- Upastha (genitals) — for reproduction
- Vak (mouth) — for speech

What are other three subtle sense organs?

Our Manas (mind), Ahamkara (ego) and Buddhi (intellect) are other three subtle sense organs. These are not creating their impressions or stimulus but also influencing our understanding and experience

through other sense organs too. Through these three we are continually manipulating or experiencing things from our perspective or mind, ego and intellect.

How to practice Pratyahara?

Pratyahara of cognitive and action senses can be practised easily employing relaxation, holding still, closing eyes or ears, removing or keeping away from all the situations where we were receiving negative food or intake through all these sense organs. Our mind can be focussed on a point, thought or idea, as we have many jnana yoga and relaxation techniques. Refining our mind, letting go of old habits and selfishness can help practising ego-pratyahara. Also, selfless service is one of the best tools to master ego-pratyahara. Buddhi pratyahara can be practised through contemplating on universal ideas and divine nature.

What is Dharna?

Once you have mastered your mind and senses, then you got them under your perfect control. You need to learn and master how to focus or concentrate your mind on one point. Your conscious effort to focus on one point is known as Dharana, the sixth limb in Yoga. Maharishi Patanjali states that "concentration is ability or skill of mind." This means we need to train our mind to be able to focus on one point.

III. 1 Desa bandhas cittasya dharana,
Dharana is unifying, focusing, collecting, and binding together (bandha) the consciousness principle that exists in mind (cittasya) and then focusing it (bandha) upon an object (Desa). The place (Desa) can be internal (Antar) or external (Bahya) or it can be very subtle (Suksma) or secret (Gupta).

How can breath be used a Dharna?

Try to sit straight with the spine erect. Hold your hands on your knees in Jnana Mudra and softly close your eyes. Now focus your mind in the middle of your nostrils and try to watch every in and outgoing breath. Do not allow any breath to enter in or go out without noticing is like a 'dutiful guard'. If thoughts are arousing, let them go, do not allow your mind to flow with them. Keep coming back to your breath again and again. In few days of practice, you will be able to focus your mind on your breath. This is known as concentration.

What is Samayama Yoga?

The first five limbs- Yama, Niyama, Asana, Pranayama, and Pratyahara, are also known as Bahiranga or external yoga. The last three limbs Dharana, Dhyana and Samadhi together are known as Samayama Yoga or higher yoga. These three limbs are not something we can practice, and these are states we attain through mastering the first five limbs.

What is Dhyana?

When a Yogi trains and masters the mind to be focused on one external or internal point, it brings the power of continuous flow of energy or awareness to that point. This state is known as Dhyana or meditation. When this state of meditation becomes very intense, there will be no external perception and it remains in an unbroken undisturbed meditation on the point of concentration and its meaning, this state in known as Samadhi.

How important is Meditation to attain Samadhi?

Importance of meditation can be understood by following verse of Yoga Sutra -

I. 39 Yathabhimata-dhyanad va
Samadhi can be attained from an agreeable, suitable, and customised meditation (dhyana) as one is drawn to (abhimata).

II 11. Dhyana-heyas tad-vrttayah
Meditation (dhyana) is the competent practice that annihilates (heyas) these fractures, limitations, hindrances, agitations, and turmoil's of consciousness (cit-vrtti).

Can I Practice Dhyana?

No. This path to Meditation and Samadhi begins with refining our mind and energy through Hatha Yoga. Then one learns to withdraw the senses and mind from the external world to the internal, which is known as Pratyahara. Once we can do that, then we can try to focus or concentrate our mind on one point or truth which can be external or internal. By regular practice we will come to the point that we have mastered our concentration and our mind is engaged at that point for some time, this becomes Dharana or concentration. When this single-pointed concentration lasts for an extended period, our mind becomes merged into the point of focus, that state is Dhyana or meditation.

What are three essential principals behind meditation?

We hear a sound, its one of the perception. First, there is the external vibration which is the stimulus. Second, the nerve conduction from ears that carries it to the mind. Third, the reaction from the mind, along with which arouses the knowledge of the object which was the external

cause of these different changes from the ethereal vibrations to the mental reaction. These three in Yoga are known as, Sabda (sound), Artha (meaning), and Jnana (knowledge). So by focussing on one point, when we become one with the object in single-pointed awareness, we attain meditation. Here we experience sound, meaning and knowledge of the object and these are three basic principles or quality.

What is Samadhi?

Samadhi is derived from the Sanskrit, sama, meaning "together," and dhi, meaning "mind." Samadhi is the union of our mind and awareness where our mind is not divided into many minds anymore. At any point if we reflect into our mind, we are thinking, talking, reading, watching, judging and so much more. Our mind divides into many minds. When all these minds merge back into Chitta or conscious mind, that state is known as Samadhi. Samadhi is also translated as liberation, self-realisation, enlightenment, etc.

What are kinds or types of Samadhi?

Patanjali states ten type of Samadhi. These are as follows-

1. Sabija Samadhi- In this state of the union there is still the object of concentration or meditation there. There are other four levels of samadhi under Sabija Samadhi.

1.1 Samprajnata Samadhi- In this samadhi mind attains absorption of the union in one of the four states of mind or Chitta with the support of a tool or focus point.
1.1.1 Savitarka- Union with subtle reasoning.
1.1.2 Savichara- Union with subtle thoughts.
1.1.3 Ananda- absorption or union in blissful mind.

1.1.4   Asmita- Union of wholeness or completeness of mind.
1.2   Asamprajnata Samadhi- This transition or further advance samadhi compare to Samprajnata where Sadhaka even loses the identity of concentration itself.
1.2.1   Nirvitarka- Samadhi free of reason
1.2.2   Nirvichara- Samadhi free from even subtle thoughts
1.2.3   Ananda to Asmita
1.2.4   Asmita to Nirbija
2.   Nirbija Samadhi- This Samadhi is seedless, there is no object, or I or self anymore.
3.   Dharma Megha Samadhi- Is the highest samadhi or Kaivalya, liberation, enlightenment and self-realisation.

Is Yoga mystic or esoteric?

Yes and No. Anything we have not experience or beyond the experience of our gross mind and senses is known to mystic and or esoteric. But in reality, yoga is scientific and experiential. If you can sincerely do your sadhana and follow all the practices, you can attain all the states of yoga and experience them for yourself, but until then yes they are mystic.

Is Yoga Scientific then?

Yes. Yoga is the pure spiritual science of self, divine and nature. The only difference between our modern science and yoga science is their approach to experimentation. Yoga science provides all the tried and tested tools of asana, pranayama, mudra, universal principles, energy concepts and idea. But unlike modern science, one needs to take them sincerely and practice regularly with faith for a long time to find the truth and individual experience. Swamiji Dr Gitananda Giriji mentions that yoga is the mother of the all the sciences.

What is Karma?

Karma means action, deeds or what we do. Here we need to understand that Karma is not only what we do physically, but also our mental, emotional and spiritual actions in forms of thoughts, feelings and emotions, followed by words, speech and physical activities are accounted as Karma.

We are also responsible for Karma we encourage, discourage and pay someone else to do as well as Karma that we allow to happen or block them to happen is also accounted as our Karma at some level. All our mental, verbal and physical actions done by us, getting some else to do our allowing to happen, we are to certain degree accountable for them.

What are the types of Karma?

In the form of doing, we have three types of Karma. These are Mansika (mental), Vachika (verbal) and Dahik (physical).

Mansika Karma- All those thoughts, feelings, emotions, desires, drive forces and Chitta Vrittis are classified as Manasika Karma. Our Mental actions gradually manifest into Verbal actions. Our mental karma has a significant role in individual happiness or suffering as how we deal and process each stimulus or situation in life.

Vachika Karma- This form of Kamra includes what we speak, write and communicate with others through words. We can hurt or heal someone with our words more than anything else.

Dahik Karma- Is all our actions done by employing our body, like gardening, writing, walking, caring, cooking, working, etc.

What are the types of Karma in reference to time and fruits?

There are four types of Karma in reference to past, present and future. These are

Sanchita Karma- Karma that is stored with us, or being accumulated from our past Karmas.

Prarbhdha Karma- These are Karma which is resulting or fruiting now.

Agami Karma- It is Karma that we end up doing in future, will fruit in future from all the present Karma we are doing.

Vartamana Karma- There are instant karma or actions, we do now. These may be resulting now or changing into Sanchita Karma.

Can I be free of doing Karma?

No. As Lord Krishna explains no one can be free from doing Karma all the while we are alive. We are breathing, thinking, eating, feeling, resting, sitting, walking, talking, working and all that counts under our Karma.

How can I be free from fruits of Karma?

Lord Krishna explains that only way to be free of Karma is by doing the selfless action (Niskama Karma) and he also further says offer all your efforts to divine cause or reason.

How to know what is right and wrong in Karma?

We are living in different states of mind, society and lifestyles and what may be right for one person might be wrong for someone else. Vedanta details three fundamental self-enquiry questions to find out what is right for us when we are taking karma or making a choice. These are –

1. Am I happy to accept the fruits?
2. How would it influence my family, friends and society?
3. Does it help me to attain health, happiness and spiritual growth?

If we answer yes to all three, then it should be right choice or karma at least at that moment.

What are five fundamental Truths or reality?

The five truths Divine, soul or the living entities, material, nature and time are all eternal. The five basic facts are:
1. Isvara- the Supreme Power
2. Jiva- the living entities
3. Prakriti- the Nature
4. Karma- all physical, mental and emotional activities
5. Kala- the Time

What are the Obstacles or Antarayas on Path of Yoga?

The Sanskrit word 'Antaraya' is translated as hindrances or obstacle here, which means "to come between." Thus Antarayas move toward or come in between to produce a gap or interval in our Yoga Sadhana or Practice. In classical yoga, Antarayas are physical, mental, emotional, emotional and attitude problems or disturbances comes face to face in our yogic evolutionary process.

What are Nine Obstacles?

Probably the best-known traditional obstacles are the nine listed in the first chapter of the Yoga-Sutra (1.30). The first, sickness (vyadhi), is a physical obstacle. The other eight are mental obstacles- languor (styana), doubt (samshaya), heedlessness (pramada), sloth (alasya), dissipation (avirati), false vision (bhranti-Darshana), nonattainment of yogic stages (alabdha-bhumikatva), and instability in these stages (anavasthitatva).

What are the four tools to remove obstacles?

Faith- in the righteousness of what you are doing as well as in your strength or ability to attain the success in your yoga path will keep motivating you in moments of distractions. "The person who has control over himself attains success verily through faith; none other can succeed. Therefore, with faith, the Yoga should be practised with care and perseverance." (Shiva-Samhita)

Intention- Your clear intention and constant mindfulness (smirti) of what and why you are doing regarding both short-term and long-term goals and the subtle adjustments of everyday practice will help you to prevent as well as prepare to deal with the obstacles.

Contentment (Santosha)- Being realistic and accepting both success and failure with grace, and self-respect; and also willingness to take risks and embrace uncertainty will prevent you from disappointment. "As long as one is not satisfied in the self, he will be subjected to sorrow. With the rise of contentment, the purity of one's heart blooms. The contented man who possesses nothing owns the world." (Yoga-Vashishtha)

Discrimination (Viveka)- Carefully discriminating (Viveka) between what's right and wrong your yoga sadhana as well as what is important what is not and avoiding them will keep you safe from obstacles.

Swadhyaya- awareness of body, mind, and emotions can keep you notified about ongoing or upcoming obstacles as well as their results. "By listening to instructions, by contemplation and by being in the company of a calm and sure-minded preceptor, doubts can be removed." (Shiva-Samhita)

What are five states of mind?

Our mind has five states from very disturbed to entirely focused. Depending on the degree of distraction, Yoga philosophy categorises the mind under five stages of being:

- Kshipta or disturbed,
- Mudha or stupefied,
- Vikshipta or distracted,
- Ekagra or focused, one pointed and
- Niruddha or the entirely balanced state of mind.

What are Five modifications of Mind or Pancha Vrittis?

Yoga categorises thoughts or mental modifications in five categories. These are the cause of klishta/bad and aklishta/good in our life; pain and pleasure, suffering and joy. These are:

1. Pramana – Pramana is our direct real knowledge or experience directly, through scriptures or realised masters.
2. Viparyaya - Unreal cognition, or experiencing what is not real like seeing a snake in a rope in the dark.
3. Vikalpa -Imagination. T
4. Nidra - Deep sleep.
5. Smriti- Memory, and recalling what we experienced in the past.

What are Pancha Kleshas or cause of suffering?

According to Patanjali, "there are five kinds of mental impressions, afflictions, or modifications (kleshas):
1) ignorance- not knowing the truth or ignoring the truth (avidya),
2) I-ness, individuality, or egoism (asmita),
3) attachment or addiction to mental impressions or objects (raga),
4) aversion to thought patterns or objects (dvesha),
5) clinging to life or objects for any cost as well as fear of loss or death."

What are the subtle four remedies?

These are Maitri (friendliness), Karuna (kindness, compassion), Mudita (cheerfulness) and Upeksha (living in equanimity and letting go).

What is Abhyasa?

Swamiji Dr Gitananda Girji mentions his 3Rs for success in Raja Yoga as Abhyasa, which means doing your practice, again and again with awareness, dedication and faith. These are REGULARITY, RYTHM, and REPETITION.

Doing our sadhana, following your practice every day, in the timescale we are instructed or meant to practice. Rhythm or harmony in practice also intensify it, makes it exciting and fruitful instead of dull and boring.

We cant just practice yoga for few hours a week to achieve mastery. I have seen lots of people doing fasting for a day and live on junk and unhealthy food for rest of the month. Repetition is also essential. We learn so many practices, methods and choose to practice different practices every day. In yoga, each tool and practice needs to be practiced for a certain time period. This will bring some experience or achievement in your sadhana, which brings encouragement, and enthusiasm.

What is Vairagya?

Vairagya is a Sanskrit term meaning "detachment." It is a state of being free of attachment to material and non-material aspects of life. It can also be defined as the mental state of mind that lets go of all affections and its attraction or desires towards any sort of pleasure and focus on finding joy or pleasure in union with the divine. Letting go of feelings such as pride, ego, aversion, inferiority and superiority complex, false identities and fear, are all also associated with vairagya.

What are three Gunas?

According to Ayurveda; medicines and foods are sattvic, rajasic or tamasic or a combination of these gunas. The gunas are three fundamental attributes that represent the natural evolutionary process through which the subtle becomes gross. In turn, gross objects, by action and interaction among themselves, may again become subtle.

Thus the three gunas are defined as:
Sattva : Essence (subtle)
Rajas: Activity
Tamas: Inertia (gross)

What is Pancha Mahabhutas?

The Pancha-Mahabhutas / The Five Elements: A further manifestation of Prakriti is five elements. This whole physical world, living and non-living materials are created by their different composition.

Pancha Mahabhutas / Five Elements

Akash	Agni	Vayu	Jala	Prithvi
Ether / Space	Fire	Air	Water	Earth

These are:
- Akash/space as we experience in the subtle world, also known as ether.
- Vayu / Air (From Akash emerges Vayu/ air)
- Agni / Fire (then Agni emerges)
- Jala/ water (then Jala)
- Prithvi / Earth (the last to emerge)

What is Pranava?

Pranava, also known as AUM is the most sacred mantra in Yoga and Hinduism. It is known as 'cosmic or divine sound'. It is the closest sound vibration to the sound of universal mother creative force or divine energy.

How do I chant a Mantra?

A mantra can be chanted loud, known as Vachika Jap or loud verbal chanting. Second, you can chant mantra as Mansa Japa, means reciting the mantra in your mind. Third, you can chant Bhava Japa, means feeling the vibration of mantra and its meaning. This is also known as Ajapa-Japa. Mantra has three essential parts- chanting, knowing its purpose if possible and experiencing the vibration.

What are Guru and Sadguru?

Guru means a teacher or guide who can lead from darkness to light. Guru or Sadguru is generally used in the context of a spiritual master or guide who can show us the path to self-realisation.

How important is it to use Sanskrita in Yoga?

Sanskrita is one of most ancient and scientific language based on vibration and essence of each word and syllable used. It is a scholarly language used for all the Hindu and Yogic scripture to keep things scientific, simple and precise. It word used in Sanskrita will have its vibration to channel the energy in various naris, activate or open various chakras and stimulate various parts of the brain. So more you use the Sanskrita better it is for your Sadhana, health and well being.

How do I attain success in Yoga?

You can attain success in Yoga by regular practice, dedication, faith, enthusiasm and simplicity. Live a simple and moderate life.

Which are Three Bandhas?

Bandha means a lock or bond. Hatha Yoga describes three bandhas to awaken our seed potential energies and purify associated chakras. These three are as follows-

Moola bandha- Anal and perineum area.
Uddiyana Bandha- Abdominal lock
Jalandhara Bandha- Throat lock.

What is a mudra?

Mudra means a gesture or expression of energy. Mudras are used in Hatha Yoga to channel energy in various parts of our body, brain, chakras and naris to purify, enhance and activate those areas, so prana can flow freely from Mooladhara to Sahashrara, leading to self-realisation. Mudras are therapeutic energy work and can help healing our body, mind and soul.

Do I need to live extreme ascetic life to be successful in Yoga?

No. Yoga advises us to live a moderate life. Lord Krishna in Bhagavata explains it very beautifully. He says "one who overeats or starve too much, one who sleeps too much or not sleeping enough, one who is not doing anything or one who is overdoing it, will never attain success in yoga."

Is Yoga Kriya or Akriya?

Kriya means doing, changing or moving while Akriya means not doing, or stable. First five limbs (Yama, niyama, asana, pranayama and pratyahara) are yoga kriyas while last three limbs (dharna, Dhyana and samadhi) are akriya yoga as these are states of experience or being and not doing.

Do I need to follow a particular path or lineage of Yoga?

You don't have to, but it is better to follow a particular path once you have found that one you feel or understand that it is providing you all the tools and practices you need to follow to attain success in your goal. But until then you have to follow and try many paths with your conscience and discrimination or Viveka.

What are Avidya and Vidya?

Avidya means lack of knowledge or ignorance. In yoga, ignorance is not only not knowing but also denying the facts or truth we know.

Vidya is knowledge or wisdom. It is not only what we know but also what we have experienced for ourselves. In yogic and spiritual context Vidya knows the Truth, Reality about Self, Higher Self, their Nature, and Universal laws of creation, evolution and involution.

What is Satsanga?

Satsanga is a Sanskrit term meaning "the company or association with truth or truth seekers" or "companionship of righteous or virtuous". It further references as spending time with like-minded people to discuss spiritual thoughts, ideas and experiences.

The word Satsanga has two root words, sat means truth and sanga, mean "companionship", and therefore, satsanga can also be state of mind and thoughts in friendliness (maitri) with Truth and Reality or Divine.

In the Spiritual level, Satsang is associated with the inner quality of sattva (goodness or purity), one of the three qualities of nature (Prakriti). Sattva manifests as thoughtfulness, knowledge, peace and contemplation. A sattvic person makes a natural satsangi, or "seeker of truth." Satsanga is one of the easiest and quickest paths to attain Samadhi or Self-realisation.

What is Kirtan?

Kirtan is the call-and-response form of chanting and singing of Mantras and devotional bhajans or songs. Kirtan is the joyful way to sing devotional songs, spiritually uplifting songs, prayers or sacred names of divine-like Krishna, Shiva, Aum, Guru, Ganesh, Durga, and many more names of supreme consciousness. It is accompanied with traditional Indian instruments such as the mrdanga (drum) and kartalas (hand cymbals), harmonium, sitar, veena, etc. Kirtan is powerful singing and chanting path of Sanatana Dharma and yoga to evoke supreme consciousness.

There are many different forms of kirtan, and there are many melodies based on classical Indian notes to help transcend the minds of the partaker into divine consciousness and help them connect with own true divine self. Mantras and devotional songs with instruments and joyfulness help to engage our mind and senses to lead them into natural Nada Meditation.

What is Bhajan?

Bhajan is a Sanskrit word meaning "singing or praising qualities of the divine." It is also the term used for Hindu devotional songs, devoted to various aspects or qualities of the divine.

The term covers a wide range of devotional music, from a simple mantra, few verses on quality, name or praise in any form of divine and the more complex once. Typical Bhajans are lyrical, easy to follow and convey love for the Divine. It can gradually lead us to experience inner sounds of divine quality in us, awake chakras and kundalini. Bhajans are sung in call-response form.

What are Puja and Aarti?

Puja or aarti is the act of showing love and devotion to a form of divine, a spirit, or any aspect of the divine, deities, god one believes in through invocations, prayers, songs, and rituals. An essential part of puja for the Hindu devotee is making a spiritual connection with the divine. Most often that contact is facilitated through an object: an element of nature, a sculpture, a vessel, a painting, or a print. Puja or aarti is followed by taking blessings from fire to bring purity, change and prosperity. This is followed by putting a simple white dot for peace and red dot for bravery, light and enthusiasm in life.

What is Namaskar or Namaste?

Namaskar is a respectful greeting gesture used by Indians and Yoga followers. Namah in Sanskrita means salutation, greeting and it also means not me, egoless, and Kar means I do or offer. So namaskar is an egoless, I-less greeting or salutations. It commonly and spiritually translated as "soul or self in me is greeting to self on the soul in you." Namaste is more traditional greeting in the form of Mudra or gesture to express our respect, gratitude and greeting to the spirit in others with

joining our hands together to heart with chin little down as if you are looking into the heart.

Why do we traditionally touch the feet of a Guru or Master in Yoga?

It is common practice among Hindus and Indians to touch feet of their elders, teachers, spiritual masters or Gurus and respected once. It is a way to express that I let go my ego, I am here, seeking, and praying for your guidance, blessings and love to grow in my own life. Touching the feet is a way to express that "I am humble, grateful to you. That, I am here to serve you, because I have faith and trust in myself as I am ready to receive your wisdom, blessings, knowledge. Also, I have faith in you that you can help me to learn, practice, grow and attain my true potentiality in this life. Many seekers also use offerings in the form of flowers, clothes, fruits, and other offerings to express this gratitude.

Is there a Scientific explanation of touching feet?

The nerves from our brain spread across all your body. These nerves or wires end in the fingertips of our hand and feet. When we touch the fingertips of our hand to those of their feet, a circuit is immediately formed, and the energies of two bodies are connected. Our fingers and palms are receivers and feet, and toes are giver ends of energy.

What is Mauna?

Mauna is a Sanskrit term meaning "silence," which is one of very important sadhana or Practice in Sanatana Dharma and yoga. In yoga, practising silence while meditating, performing asanas, doing karma yoga, eating food is a simple way of removing distractions and preserving our subtle pranic energies. This allows the mind to focus entirely on practice, subject or whatever we are doing to achieve the enhanced state of

concentrated mind. Mauna translates as 'not-speaking', but in the true sense, silence is also not communicating in form and gradually even the inner silence of mind.

What is Vrata?

The term Vrata comes from the Sanskrit root vr, meaning "rule," "conduct", "discipline", or "restraint," and rta means "order", "oath," or "to follow with own will". Vrata in generally used for spiritual practice, custom, rule or observance. In yoga a sadhaka makes his rules or guidelines on his own or under the guidance of his Guru to succeed in mastering his body and mind, leading to Samadhi. It is an act of faith, devotion and dedication in practices.

What is Yoga Therapy?

Yoga Therapy is adapted, modified or applied aspects of Asana, kriya, pranayama, visualisation and relaxation techniques to help prevent, heal, or rehabilitation of people with many health issues. Yoga has proved to significantly helpful in all the stress-related disorders, mental and emotional problems.

Dr Ananda Balayogi Bhavanani, ICYER, India in Yoga Chikitsa book writes that "Yoga as a mode of therapy (Yoga Chikitsa) has become extremely popular and a great number of studies and systematic reviews offer scientific evidence of its potential in treating a wide range of psychosomatic conditions. Yoga understands health and well-being as a dynamic continuum of human nature and not merely a 'state' to be reached and maintained. Yoga helps the individual to establish sukha sthanam which may be defined as a dynamic sense of physical mental and spiritual well-being."

According to our Guru Yogamaharishi Dr Swami Gitananda Giri Guru Maharaj, "Yoga Chikitsa is virtually as old as Yoga itself. Indeed, the

'return of mind that feels separated from the Universe in which it exists' represents the first Yoga therapy. Yoga Chikitsa could be termed "man's first attempt at Unitive understanding of mind-emotions-physical distress and is the oldest holistic concept and therapy in the world."

TKV Desikachar and Kausthub Desikachar explains that "Yoga therapy is a self-empowering process, where the care-seeker, with the help of the Yoga therapist, implements a personalized and evolving Yoga practice, that not only addresses the illness in a multi-dimensional manner but also aims to alleviate his/her suffering in a progressive, non-invasive and complementary manner. Depending upon the nature of the illness, Yoga therapy can not only be preventative or curative, but also serve a means to manage the illness, or facilitate healing in the person at all levels."

What is Adhi-Vyadhi?

In Anandamaya Kosha, a man is healthiest with perfect harmony and balance of all his faculties. At Vijnanamaya Kosha, there are movements but are channelised in the right direction. As such, it is in the Manomaya Kosha; the imbalances start, says the yoga texts. These imbalances amplify themselves resulting in mental illnesses called " Adhis ". At this stage, there are no symptoms at the physical level. Prompted by the perpetual growth of desires, these mental diseases concealed in us, begin to manifest themselves externally and gradually if we don't heal them at the time they take roots in our mind-body. They create the imbalance in our Pranamaya Kosha which manifests in the body in the form of physical problems known as Vyadhi or Diseases. Adhi-Vyddhi is the ancient concept which now modern medicine and psychology are explaining regarding psycho-somatic or stress-related health problems.

What is Moksha?

Moksha is the concept of ultimate freedom and liberation from birth cycles of cycle birth, life and death. Once one attains Moksha, they would not have to return to human body anymore to go through Maya, illusion and suffering. Moksha comes from Sanskrita root 'muc' meaning 'to free', it frees the individual from its bondage with body, mind, and karma. To attain moksha one has to reach absolute freedom, peace and oneness with the Divine.

What is a Siddhi?

Siddhi is the Sanskrita or Yogic term used for spiritual or mystical powers and abilities through dedicated yoga sadhana or practices. Siddhi is fruit, accomplishment, or success in your tasks taken. In Yoga, Patanjali defines them as milestones and not the result. Patanjali further warns that "don't ever get stuck into them as they bring ego, power, and fame".

Siddhis are generally powers which can enable you to control your body and mind. You may be able to read minds, see beyond everyone's sight, hear what no else can hear. You may be able to see the past and future.

What is a Yogi?

A Yogi is one who has mastered his body and mind and has attained Samadhi or self-realisation where self-has become with the higher self.

What is a Sadhu?

A Sadhu is a Hindu or Yoga ascetic who has left all material attachments with his will and dedicated his life to achieving spiritual liberation, or moksha. They usually wear distinctive clothing (orange robs) as a

symbol of their sannyasa, which is a Hindu term for renunciation. The female equivalent of a sadhu is a Sadhvi.

What is a Siddha?

Lord Krishna explains that one who has mastered his/her mind and never deviates from its single-pointed concentration due to all the worldly attractions or aversions is Siddha or Master.

Is Yoga to Control our Mind?

No. Patanjali mentions that "yoga is still or quietening whirlpools of mind- Yoga-Chitta-vritti-norodah". Yoga is a state or goal to be achieved through all its Kriyas and Prikriyas, concepts and ideas to purify our body, mind, sense, and ego to attain the state of still or focused mind.

What is Ananda, Parmananda, and Satchidananda?

Ananda means joy or blissful state or experience. Ananda in generally used as a positive emotion of happiness. Parmananda means highest or divine form of joyfulness or happiness. This is absolute bliss or joy which we experience in higher states of meditation. Sat means 'Truth or Reality', and Chit means 'consciousness or pure mind' while Ananda means 'joy or bliss'. Satchidananda is state of experience of joyfulness when our mind or awareness attains self-realisation, truth or reality.

Who is Adhikari In Yoga?

In yoga one who is genuinely desiring or seeking to learn, practice and follow the path of yoga to attain Samadhi, Union, health and well being is known as Adhikari of Yoga. Adhikari means one who is eligible or one who deserves.

What is Guru Dakshina?

Guru means one who guides us on the path of self-realisation or success in Yoga. Dakshina implies to donation or offering to appreciate what we have received from someone. Guru Dakshina is one of the traditional rituals to offer, express and understands our Guru for passing his /her knowledge and guidance by offering flowers, fruits, money, clothes, etc. in any way we can afford.

What is Diksha?

Diksha is another Yogic and Hindu practice or ritual where a Guru (the teacher) and Shishya (the student) accept spiritual relation to learn and practice together on the path of self-realisation. In many traditional ashrams, it is a fundamental practice, and Guru will teach all the higher methods after Diksha only.

What is Dvaita?

Madhvacharya, the propounder of this philosophy explains Brahman or Parmatman (higher self or divine self) and Atman (individual self) as two different entities and Bhakti as the keyPath or route to liberation. According to this philosophy, there are many Jivatma (individual soul) and only one Paramatma (divine self).

What is Advaita?

Adi Shankaracharya is known as the propagator of this Advaita Philosophy. This is the oldest branch of Vedanta. This path or philosophy explains that Brahman or Parmatman is only Reality or Truth, which is eternal. Rest of the world is illusory (Maya) and changing all the time. This Maya, illusion or ignorance is the cause of all the sufferings. Jnana

Yoga or acquiring true knowledge or attaining reality will lead us to Samadhi, where Self-attains union with the higher Self.

Shankaracharya states that "Brahma Satya Jagat mithya, jivo Brahmaiva Na aparah". Meaning Brahman (the absolute) alone is real; this world is unreal, and the jiva or the individual soul is non-different from Brahman.

What are the few of many Classical Meanings of Yoga?

1. Yoga Anushasanam means "yoga is discipline". (Patanjali)
2. Yogachitta-vritti-nirodha means "yoga is stilling or quietening whirlpools of mind". (Patanjali)
3. Yama-Niyama-...-Ashtanga-Yogah – "Yama, Niyama, Asana, Pranayama, Pratyahara, Dharna, Dhyana and Samadhi are eight limbs of Raja Yoga". (Patanjali)
4. Yoga is Samadhi or Union according to Patanjali.
5. Yoga Karmeshu Kaushalam – means "yoga is the skill in action". (Lord Krishna, Bhagavad Gita)
6. Yoga Samatvam means yoga is living with equanimity. (Lord Krishna, Bhagavad Gita)
7. Yoga is Niskama Karma -means fruitless action. Swami Gitananda Giriji says it beautifully "Do your best and leave the rest".
8. According to Swamiji Gitananda Giriji Yoga is a goal as well as a path. He states that yoga is the mother of all the sciences.

What is Naam Daan in Yoga?

Naam in Sanskrita means name. Daan means what is given to others. A Guru or teacher provide a spiritual or yogic name to his/her student as a title to help them grow further on Yogic path. It is the symbol of removing our associations with old conditionings and attachments.

What is Dharma?

Dharma means duty or responsibility we need to fulfil. We all are born in this life to meet particular dharma to learn and experience lessons to grow further on the path of evolution. Lord Krishna mentions in Bhagavat Gita that it is essential for us all to follow our dharma or do our duties to our best we can.

How can I attain success in yoga or any other goals in life?

Swamiji Dr Gitananda Giriji mentions 3R's for success in our life. These three R's are -REGULARITY, RHYTHM, REPETITION. We all need to follow our practices, duties and dharmas regularly, repeat them over and over again and find the rhythm to enjoy them.

What is Mitahara?

From Sanskrit, Mita means "moderate", and Ahara means "diet" or "food consumption." Mitahara in practice means moderate, healthy dietary habots, where you eat enough to be healthy. Overeating or starving our body are considered obstacles in Yoga Sadhana.

Do I need to follow yoga practices extreme intensively to be successful?

Patanjali states three levels of intensity in yoga practices, Mridu (gentle), Madhya (moderate), Adhimatra (intense). He further says that success in Sadhana will depend on the level of intensity. But Lord Krishna in Bhagavad Gita advocates moderate living for success in Sadhana. He mentions that "one overeats or does not eat enough, one who sleeps too much or does not sleep enough, one who over exercise not exercising

enough, will never attain success in Yoga". So simply "doing your best, with sincere effort and faith is key to success".

What is Shavasana?

Shava is a Sanskrit word, which means corpse or dead and Asana means posture or pose. Shavasana is a practice or posture in Yoga leading us to experience state where the body becomes still as in corpse. Once body attains this stillness and ease, all our pranic forces flow inward back to their source points, recharging and revitalising our body, mind and soul.

This asana stimulates the Mooladhara (root) Chakra because the entire base of the body is in contact with the earth. Energizing this chakra through Shavasana leads to grounding the individual, providing the inner stability and vitality necessary for higher meditative practices in yoga.

What is Yoga Nidra?

Yoga is Union or mindfulness, while Nidra means sleep. Yoga Nidra is conscious sleep. Yoga Nidra techniques are used to channel our mind and vital forces to enhance the quality of life forces. Yoga Nidra can help to charge, healing and to rejuvenate our body and mind.

Does Brahmacharya mean complete abstain from sex?
No. Brahamachariya means living our lives in harmony with all the natural forces. Yoga promotes growth in four phases. Second stage or ashram is Grihastha, where we make family, and hence Brahamachariya cannot mean complete abstain from sex. It is more control and discipline of our sensual energy and desires. Vedanta explains that we should never suppress our desires. We should learn how to fulfil them or transcend them to attain health, happiness and grow spiritually.

What are key four Asanas?

Hatha Yoga mentions 84,00,000 asanas, and further, it says that 84 are more significant. Out of the four are most important. These four are Dhyana-Asanas or postures for meditation. These are-

Sukhasana- Simply sitting cross-legged in the relaxed pose.

Vajrasana or Bhadrasana- Sitting on your heels in kneeling position.

Padmasana- Lotus pose where you place your feet on top of thighs close to the pelvis.
Siddhasana- Placing one heel against the perineum above the anus and another heel on top of the first one as if you are hiding your genitals. This is known as Perfect Pose.

What is Ahara Vihara?

Ahara means food or what we feed to our body, mind and soul. Ahara includes food we eat and drink. Ahara also means all the intake of sense organs. Ahara for our mind and brain is also what we read, watch, and listen.
Vihara means lifestyle or what we do. Vihara includes all our physical activities, habits, work, exercise and all that we do as part of life.

How is Ahara Vihara concept important for health and well-being?

Ahara is food for body, mind and soul, while Vihara is our lifestyle. Our Ahara-vihar is representing who we are in the real sense. If we are eating unhealthy and junk food, our body will become weak and toxic. We lose our health and well-being. Similarly, a positive lifestyle with balanced diet, exercise, rest, work, entertainment, family and social time, etc.

all have the positive effect on our health and well-being. As Swami Gitananda Giriji mentions "Health and Happiness are our birth rights, but we all need to claim them by doing everything that leads us to health and happiness".

What is Aura?

The aura is an electromagnetic energy field that surrounds our body. In a healthy person, this energy is egg-shaped or oval energy that encompasses the body. This aura is like glow or radiance of our body-mind-energy together. The colour of aura can be different in same person depending on their body and mind states. The aura consists of seven levels/layers/auric bodies, also known as the physical, astral, lower, higher, spiritual, intuitional, and absolute planes. The colours of aura also affect a person's feelings, emotions, thought patterns, behaviour, and overall health.

What is Atman -Parmatman?

Atman is individual soul, while Parmatman means Higher or the universal soul. If Parmatman is ocean, then Atman can be represented by a drop of water in it. Like the sea does not exist without a drop of water or drop becomes ocean once it finds union back within it; similarly, Atman and Parmatman are one. Dr Ananda explains beautifully that Atman becomes individual soul when it is attached with Chitta-vrittis, ego and Asmita.

What is Jiva?

Jiva means life or soul. This is another term being used for individual soul or atman. Many schools used the name Jiva or Life for individual soul bonded by karma, ego and I-ness.

What is Prakriti?

Prakriti in Yoga and Hinduism refers to a primal creative or natural force behind all that manifests. Prakriti also represents all the essential qualities of all the materials and non-materials that exist. The term is derived from the Sanskrit Pra, meaning "beginning," and Kriti, meaning "creation."

Prakriti is composed of three Gunas :
1. Creation (rajas)
2. Preservation (sattva)
3. Destruction (tamas)

What are six vital Indian Philosophies?

Indian Philosophy, or in Sanskrit, Darshanas, refers to any of several traditions of philosophical thought that originated in the Indian subcontinent. These six primary schools of philosophies are followed by most Hindus in one or other form. These are various practical ways of living life to attain Self-realisation. These six are Samkhya, Yoga, Nyaya, Vaisheshika, Purva Mimamsa and Vedanta.

What is Samkhya Darshana?

Samkhya is the oldest of the Indian philosophical systems, and it explains that everything in reality evolutes from Purusha (self or soul) and Prakriti (matter, creative force or energy in the cause of all creation). It is a based on Dvaita or dualist system where self and matter are seen attached. By realising that Purusha is free from all the matter and changes, one attains Self-realisation.

What is Yoga Darshana?

The Yoga Darshana or Philosophy compiled by Patanjali as Yoga Sutras accepts Samkhya. This provides the more practical approach of Ashtanga Yoga to free the self from Chitta-vrittis, their outcomes and sufferings. Yoga believes in Purusha, or Individual soul has the potential to become Divine or Higher Self, Isvara.

What is Nyaya Darshana?

The Nyaya school is based on the Nyaya Sutras, written by Aksapada Gautama. Its methodology is based on a system of logic that has subsequently been adopted by the majority of the Indian schools. Its followers believe that obtaining valid knowledge or wisdom (Jnana - the four sources of which are direct experience, inference, reasoning and testimony) is the only way to attain freedom from suffering and pain.

What is Vaisheshika Darshana?

Kanada founded the Vaisheshika school, and it is atomist and pluralist in nature. The basis of the school's philosophy is that all objects in the physical universe are reducible to a finite number of atoms, and Brahman is known as the fundamental force behind the consciousness in these atoms. The Vaisheshika and Nyaya schools eventually merged because of their closely related metaphysical theories. Vaisheshika explains that perception and inference are sources of valid knowledge.

What is Purva Mimamsa Darshana?

The Purva Mimamsa school is based on faith In Vedas and following all the rituals and practices explained in them. It advocates performing fire-ceremonies or Yjanas to attain health and well-being.

What is Vedanta Darshana?

The Vedanta, or Uttara Mimamsa, school concentrates on the philosophical teachings of the Upanishads (mystic or spiritual contemplations within the Vedas), rather than the Brahmanas (instructions for ritual and sacrifice). The Vedanta focus on meditation, self-discipline and spiritual connectivity, more than traditional ritualism.

What are six sub-schools or branches of Vedanta?

Due to the mysterious, complex and poetic nature of the Vedanta Sutras, the school separated into six sub-schools, each interpreting the texts in their ways. These are

Advaita – Atman or soul and Brahman or supreme soul are one.
Visishtadvaita – Supreme Being has a definite name, form, qualities, like Vishnu.

Dvaita- Believes in separate realities of Soul, Higher Soul and Matter.

Dvaitadvaita – This explains that the Supreme Soul is independent, but soul and matter are dependent.

Shuddhadvaita – This believes that Lord Krishna is the highest or absolute form of Higher-Self.

Achintya Bheda Abheda- the soul, is both distinct and non-distinct from Krishna or Divine Self.

What is Isvara or Divine in Yoga?

Isvara is often mistranslated with the English term, "God". Isvara specifically is not atheistic idea (as yoga is not theistic). In other

words, the word Isvara specifically refers to the formless and deity-less, "aspectless aspect" of the divine aspect of Reality in Yoga. The word, Isvara, thus expresses or symbolises completeness, the whole or infinite mind and as such cannot be represented by symbols being the nothingness that includes everything. It is that individual Purusha who is free from all that is influencing it otherwise. So we all have potential to attain Divinity.

Following four verse of yoga sutra clarify all the misleading thoughts regarding the Isvara-

Klesha-karma-vipakasayair apara-mrshta purusa-visesa Isvara (Sutra 24)
Isvara is the purest (a-para-mrshta) aspect (visesa) of pure undifferentiated universal consciousness (purusa) which is untouched and unaffected by taint (klesha), karma, and the seed-germs (asayair) that result (vipaka) from common desire and propensities.

Tatra-nir-atishayam Sarvajna-bijam(Sutra 25)

There (Tatra) [isvara] is the seed and origin (bija) of absolute (nir-atishayam), unsurpassed, and complete omniscience (Sarvajna).

Tasya vachakah Pranava(Sutra 27)

Isvara is expressed and represented (vachakah) by the vibratory energy contained in the Pranava (the sacred syllable, om).

What is Yajna or Yagya?

Yajna is a Hindu ceremony or ritual using Agni Deva or Fire God as the medium or channel to worship or invoke various aspects of Divine forces. Generally Yajnas are performed to bless various aspects of life and showing our gratitude through various offerings to the Fire God.

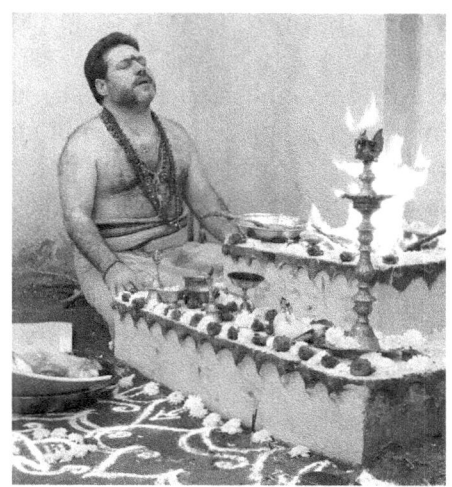

Dr Ananda Balayogi performing Yajna at Ananda Ashram, Puducherry

Why are English Sanskrita words spell differently in different texts?

Sanskrita is a phonetic language and hence people use various English syllables to help their readers to understand the actual sounds the way they are hearing it. Dialects may also be taken into account for example; in North India you may hear (for yoga) 'Yog', while in south you will hear 'Yogaha'.

What is Ahamkar?

Ahamkara is literally translated as Ego. Ego in western culture can be seen as something negative as part of our personality. Ego is that general casual force or energy which makes us to think, believe, act and react in a certain way. Our ego influences all our perceptions and experiences.

Do I have to kill my Ego?

No. There are many ways to classify our ego. The easiest and general way we understand two types of ego- positive or constructive ego, and negative or destructive ego. Ego can also be seen as selfish or self-centred where 'I' becomes more important than anything else, and then humanistic or self-less ego, which leads us to do things for the benefit of humanity and others. In the beginning we need to refine our ego, to let go all the negativity and grow a positive ego, which can lead us to follow righteousness.

What is the role of Ego in our Yogic evolution?

Our Ego or Ahamkara has a key role in our evolution. Just remember ego is one of the essential forces which gets us to move forward and act on things and plan to achieve the goal. We need a positive and strong ego to wake up and do our Sadhana. We need that ego-force to help us go out to learn and teach. Ego-less people generally tend to live a goal-less or aimless life. While spiritual self-realisation is highest goal or aim anyone can seek or aspire to.

INDEX

Abhyasa	106
Adhi-Vyadhi	115
Adhikari	117
Advaita	118
Agami Karma	102
Ahamkara	128
Ahara-Vihara	122
Ahimsa	79
Ammaji on Pranayama	88
Ananda, Parmananda, Satchidananda	117
Antaranga Yoga	48
Antarayas or Obstacles	103
Aparigraha	80
Asana	77, 83,
Ashram	76
Asteya	79
Atman-Parmatman	123
Aura	123
Bahiranga Yoga	48
Bandha	109
Bhagavata Gita	64
Bhajan	112
Bhakti Yoga	60
Bhastrika Pranayama	90
Bhramari Pranayama	89
Brahmachariya	80
Chatur Ashrams	43
Chatur Dharma	43
Chatur Yoga	44, 73
Classical Asanas	84
Classical Meanings of Yoga	119

Classical Pranayamas	89
Contentment	104
Dahika Karma	101
Dharna	78, 96, 97
Dhyana	78, 97, 98
Diksha	118
Discrimination	104
Dhyana Yoga	51
Dr Swami Gitananda Giri Ji on Pranayama	92
Dvaita	118
Dvapara Yuga	74
Eight limbs or Yoga	48, 77
Endocrine System and Chakras	58
Faith	104
Five fundamental truths	103
Five Modifications of Mind	105
Five States of Mind	105
Four aspects of Pranayama	88
Four Key Asanas	122
Four Vedas	45
Four Yugas	73
Gheranda Samhita	71
Gunas	107
Guru and/or Sadguru	08
Guru Dakshina	118
Hatha Yoga	48
Hatha Yoga in Gitananda Tradition	92
Hatha Yoga Pradipika	69
Hinduism	43, 45, 46
Ida Nari	55
Intention	104
Isvara	126

Isvara Pranidhana	82
Jnana Yoga	50
Jnanendriyas	95
Kali Yuga	74
Karma	101, 102, 103
Karma Yoga	49
Karmendriyas	95
Kirtan	111
Kriya Yoga	52
Kundalini Yoga	52
Mansika Karma	101
Mantra Chant	108
Mantra Yoga	49
Mauna	113
Meditation	98
Mind and Prana	93
Mitahara	120
Moksha	116
Mudra	109
Murcha Pranayama	90
Naam Daan	119
Namaskar or Namaste	112
Naris	55
Nerve Plexus	57
Niyama	77
Nyaya Darshana	125
Pancha Kleshas	106
Pancha-Koshas	54
Pancha Mahabhutas	107
Panch Niyamas	80
Pancha Yamas	79
Pancha Vayus	86

Pancha Vayus and Chakras	87
Pancha Vrittis	105
Parampara or Lineage	59, 110
Patanjali	63
Pingala Nari	55
Plavini Pranayama.	92
Prakriti	124
Prana	85
Pranava	108
Pranayama	77, 85, 87, 93
Pranayama Kosha	55
Pranayama Yoga	52
Prarbdha Karma	102
Pratyahara	78, 94, 96
Puja and Aarti	112
Purva Mimamsa Darshana	125
Raja Yoga	47
Sadhu.	116
Samadhi	78, 99
Samayama Darshana	124
Samtosha	81
Sanchita Karma	102
Sanskrita in Yoga	109
Sata Yuga	73
Satsanga	111
Satya	79
Senses	94
Seven Chakras	53
Shaucha	80
Shata Karmas	82
Shavasana	121

Sitakari Pranayama	89
Sitali Pranayama	89
Six Indian Philosophies	124
Shiva Samhita	66
Shiva Swarodaya	69
Siddha	117
Siddhi	116
Suriya Bhedana	91
Suriya Namaskar	84
Sushumna Nari	55
Swadhyaya	81, 105
Swara Yoga	61
Tantra Yoga	50
Tapah	81
Three Bandhas	109
Treta Yuga	73
Types of Karma	101, 102
Types of Samadhi	99
Ujjayi Pranayama	91
Vachika Karma	101
Vairagya	107
Vaishashika Darshana	125
Vartaman Karma	102
Veda	44
Vedanta Darshana	126
Vidya and Avidya	110
Vijnana Bhairava Tantra	68
Vinyasa or Kriya in Hatha Yoga	84
Viveka	104
Vrata	114
Yajna	128

Yajnavalkya Samhita	72
Yama	77, 78
Yoga	42, 43, 109, 110
Yoga Chudamani	67
Yoga Darshana	125
Yoga Kriya or Akriya	110
Yoga in modern Age	85
Yoga Mysticism	100
Yoga Nidra	121
Yoga Scientific	100
Yoga Scriptures	61
Yoga Sutras	62
Yoga Therapy	114
Yoga Vashistha	65
Yogi	116

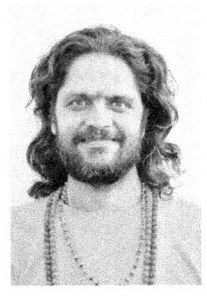
Yogachariya Jnandev
(Surender Saini)

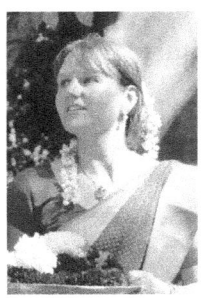
Yogacharini Deepika
(Sally Saini)

Yoga Satsanga Ashram, Wales, UK
An Authentic Yoga Teacher Training School based on Ancient Rishiculture Gitananda Yoga and Classical Hatha Yoga.

What we offer:-
Yoga Step By Step by Swamiji Dr Gitananda Giriji
Foundation course in Yoga
300hrs Yoga Teacher Training
500hrs Yoga Teacher Training
1000hrs Yoga Teacher Training
Pregnancy Yoga Teacher Training
Kids and Teens Yoga Teacher Training
Diploma in Yoga Therapy
Diploma in Yoga Philosophy

www.yogasatsanga.org